PRESCRIPTURES
For Life

Neil Elmer

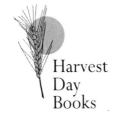
Harvest Day Books

Traverse City • Michigan

PreScriptures for Life
Copyright © 2008 by Neil Elmer

Layout and Cover Design by BookMarketingSolutions.com

Unless otherwise indicated, all Scripture references are from the American Standard Version.

All rights reserved. No part of this book may be reproduced or transmitted in any form or by any means, electronic or mechanical, including photocopying, recording, or by any information storage retrieval system without written permission from the publisher.

Published by
Harvest Day Books
an imprint of **Book Marketing Solutions, LLC**
10300 E. Leelanau Court
Traverse City, MI 49684
info@BookMarketingSolutions.com
www.BookMarketingSolutions.com

Harvest Day Books

Printed in the United States of America

Elmer, Neil.
   Prescriptures for life / Neil Elmer -- Traverse City, Mich. : Harvest Day Books, 2008.
      v. ; cm.
      ISBN: 978-0-9790834-6-4
      1. Prayer--Christianity. 2. Christianity--Prayers and devotions.
   I. Title.
BV215 .E46 2008
248.32--dc22   0807

This book is available online
at www.ReadingUp.com and www.Prescriptures.com

CONTENTS

Introduction	7
How to Use This Book	9
Essentials	16
Praying Over Children with Scripture	19
Accepting God, God's Love, and God's Presence	22
Accepting the Trustworthiness of God's Word	33
Anger, Bitterness, Hate, Resentment, and Murder	36
Blinded to the Truth of the Word	41
Character of God	50

Comfort, Contentment, Discouragement, Jealousy, Envy	55
Discernment	59
Faith	63
Faith in the Power of Jesus' Name	70
Fear and Anxiety	74
Forgiveness	88
God's Grace	95
Guilt and Shame	101
Healing, Wounds, Disease, and Injury	107
Hopelessnes, Hope, and Depression	116
Iniquity	124
Joy and Mental Stability	127
Loneliness and Feeling Forsaken	131
Love	135
Lust and Covetousness	143
Obedience, Rebellion, and God's Will and Protection	149
Our Helper: God's Spirit	161
Overcoming Evil	170

Peace and Stress	184
Prayer and Difficulty Praying	189
Pride	194
Relationships and Life: Solomon's Wisdom	203
Sorrow, Sadness, and Grief	214
Strength, Courage, and Discouragement	222
Taking All Thoughts Captive	231
Trust	238
Worry	250
Your Value, An Unloving Self-Worth, and Self-Hate	253
Psalms	261
Disease Appendix	265
About the Author	283

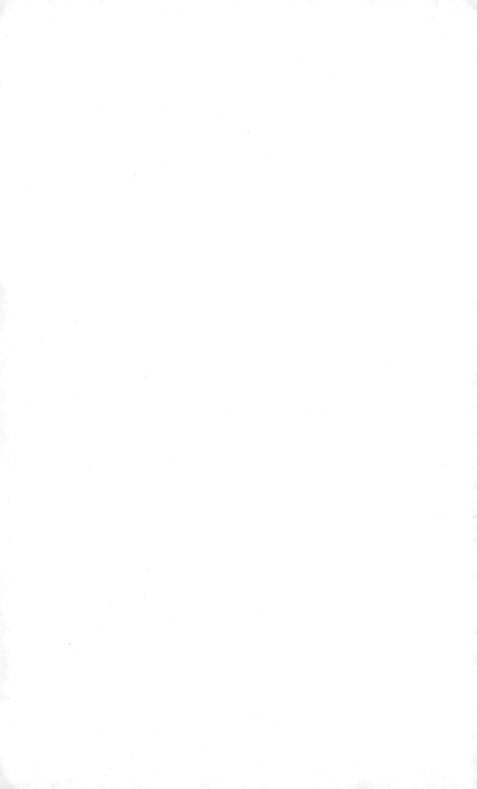

Introduction

This book is not an end-all, but rather a beginning of freedom for many. It grew from a list of scriptures and was created from the discovery that praying with scripture over people was a very powerful tool for healing. However, I felt it was clumsy to search the concordance for relevant verses while in the middle of a prayer session.

I began by developing a topical scripture prayer list. Friends then wanted these lists. And once having learned how to use the lists of scripture references, they reported how helpful they were. But they also told me they would like more verses to be included. From there, this book has evolved.

Some books are meant for entertainment, others for education or instruction. This book is intended to be used either by the reader or a friend in need. Although each topic presented could be a book in itself, the introduction to each subject area is intentionally brief and is meant to help you quickly find appropriate scripture verses. That, after all, is an important part of praying with scripture! The scripture verses found in this book are taken from the American Standard Version (ASV) of the Bible.

My greatest hope is that God's will shall be done and that many may be blessed.

How to Use This Book

This is a book about prayer. Yet it is not about all forms of prayer. This book focuses on praying with scripture verses. Although it should not be construed to mean that this is the only way to pray, this method of prayer does have a basis in scripture.

Hebrews 4:12 *For the Word of God is full of living power. It is sharper than the sharpest knife, cutting deep into our innermost thoughts and desires. It exposes us for what we really are.*

John 8:32 *and ye shall know the truth, and the truth shall make you free.*

The beauty of praying with the powerful Word of God is that another, equally powerful force comes to bear upon that prayer, and that is the Holy Spirit. We are the beneficiaries of both powers—the power of the Word and the power of the Holy Spirit—just by asking the Holy Spirit to deliver the scriptures, and the truth behind them, where they need to go.

In Luke 11:1-13, Jesus taught his disciples how to pray. Phrases such as "hallowed be thy name" have their basis in Old Testament scripture. The point I would like to make is that Jesus taught us to use scripture in prayer. Without getting into all the other aspects, this alone should be a clue. Praying with scripture is powerful! To use the scripture effectively, however, you must be in agreement with God's Word. That's the beginning of our obedience to God!

There are many who believe using scripture is such a very powerful way to pray, and it is so because these prayers are in God's will. Does that mean He decides every step of your life? No! Within His guidelines, we may have many options. If, however, we pray for something that breaks one of God's instructions for living our life, we certainly can't expect it to be answered. There may also be times when our prayers could cross the line without us realizing it. But as we grow in our relationship with God, we will come to *"know the truth, and the truth shall make you free* (John 8:32)" and we *"may be strong to apprehend with all the saints what is the breadth and length and height and depth* (Ephesians 3:18)" of Christ in us. It's guaranteed that if we are praying with scripture according to His will, we can pray with confidence.

This book will also help you to deal with strongholds of the mind. According to the original Greek translations of scripture, the mind and will are spiritual parts of our very being—that which is created in the likeness of God—and who we really are. At the disposal of our human spirit is the brain, an organ which controls the functions of our body and processes huge amounts of information. Unfortunately, some information that we have stored can be at odds with God's Word. Even when we agree logically with God's Word, at times we will act out emotionally based on the stored, faulty information.

Strongholds can be established within us in several ways. They may form through our generational line or emotional wounds we've experienced, or can even be conditioned as a result of our mother's fear during pregnancy. In any case, the mind becomes set in a certain pattern of interpreting stimuli, making it difficult for us to accurately understand events.

To clarify, let me provide two simple examples. Scripture clearly states we are all precious to God. While most Christians would agree intellectually, they may still feel they are worthless. Here's another example. We are to trust in God, yet many people live fear-filled lives, which is the opposite of trust or faith.

Let's be encouraged to be open to Jesus correcting any error that we have stored and renew our minds (see Romans 12:2). We should seek to allow the error to be rewritten with God's truth through the work of the Holy Spirit. You could think of this process as being similar to spell check on your computer. It is absolutely essential for you to agree to let Jesus work in your life, especially in hidden areas.

You may be questioning why God would want to change your mind since He created it (Ephesians 2:10). We are not talking about what God made, but rather what's in the storage container of our mind. While God may implant things into our mind and spirit, so tries His adversary. And of course, our own thoughts are there, along with memories of events of our life and interpretations of those events. So you see, we are not asking God to change our native constitution, or the way we are made, but rather, to bring His truth to replace any belief errors.

> *We are not asking God to change our native constitution, or the way we are made, but rather, to bring His truth to replace any belief errors!*

Gaining knowledge of God's Word is always appropriate. We should make this an important part of our life. But there is one thing you should consider. Even though you might memorize lots of scripture, any residual lies and distortions stored in your brain will still affect your life negatively. I believe that we must consciously allow biblical knowledge to eradicate error, otherwise we will endure increased internal conflict, stress, depression, and so forth. Allowing takes effort, obedience, and willingness to let God work in our life and to reign supreme on the throne of our heart.

Getting the junk out of our life is what God wants for us. After all, Jesus was sent to bring us out of bondage. We cannot serve Him with our unconfessed sin in the way. Praying with scripture probably won't solve all of these problems, but it may provide the foundation for moving forward.

> **Psalms 139:23-24** *23 Search me, O God, and know my heart: Try me, and know my thoughts; 24 And see if there be any wicked way in me, And lead me in the way everlasting.*

What a great way to start out our prayers—search me, lead me.

> **Hebrews 4:12-13** *12 For the word of God is living, and active, and sharper than any two-edged sword, and piercing even to the dividing of soul and spirit, of both joints and marrow, and quick to discern the thoughts and intents of the heart. 13 And there is no creature that is not manifest in his sight: but all things are naked and laid open before the eyes of him with whom we have to do.*

The Holy Spirit will do this if you ask. If you are praying for someone else, ask them if they are willing to give the Holy Spirit permission to work in their lives. The Holy Spirit may lead you to events and thoughts you need to deal with, giving you clues as to which topics to visit. You may also be led to specific scripture verses. By using this book and becoming familiar with it, you may become aware of which topics you need to turn to. If not, spend a little time reviewing the table of contents and follow your urging. When you approach the most suitable topic, do the same with specific scripture.

Many people find meditating on scripture very beneficial. That is a perfectly acceptable thing to do. The difference here is that I am suggesting you pray with scripture in a very purposeful and directed way. If you do not ask, you shall not receive.

You may still be thinking, I meditated on and studied this scripture. I really know this scripture. So why would I pray that this scripture be directed to some place in my life where there may be conflict? You may have it memorized and logically understand it, but now would be the best time to really begin to experience it. Michael Easley, the new president of Moody Bible Institute, said recently in a broadcast, "If we don't live it, then we don't really know it." These questions may help you to take a self-inventory: Are you living a completely fearless life? Do you completely trust in God for everything? If not, your fears may be holding you back.

The Apostle Peter thought he was fearless, but denied Jesus three times for fear of death. After the resurrection, while at the campfire after eating breakfast, Jesus brought truth to Peter's fear:

> **1 John 4:18** *There is no fear in love: but perfect love casteth out fear, because fear hath punishment; and he that feareth is not made perfect in love.*

So it can be understood that negative strongholds can be replaced by God's truth, which is able to set us free from the various traps we may find ourselves in. This thought deserves serious consideration. Some strongholds in our life may appear obvious, while others lie further beneath the surface. Likewise, the behavior of some people may display the turmoil raging within their heart while others prefer to conceal it.

Many people, for example, outwardly blame God for their problems and the problems of the world. They question why God caused certain circumstances to happen in their life. Some people can be downright hostile towards God. Naturally, a hostile person will have a difficult time receiving anything from God.

> *Negative strongholds can be replaced by God's truth, which is able to set us free from the various traps we may find ourselves in.*

Their heart will be hard, which means their mind will be closed.

Not so obvious are those who show no outward sign of hostility, but for some reason secretly hold God at a distance or barely put their toes in the spiritual water. In situations where a person is subconsciously angry and bitter with God, they will be blocking themselves from realizing God's love and other blessings. The antidote for anger and bitterness is forgiveness. Holding a grudge is a huge obstacle, but unforgiveness towards God may be the number one reason that people are held down.

We must learn to overcome just as Peter did—replacing fear and lies with the truth and love of God. Here's a very practical way to do that. Whenever you may be reading the Bible, or are in a Bible study, or hearing a Sunday message, and a scripture verse touches you in a special way, make a note of that verse and pray that over yourself as soon as it is convenient.

This book should be used anytime you are not at peace, or when you need something about your life to change, but it is not meant to replace anything else you are doing in Jesus' name for healing and transformation. However, this process of praying with scripture verses may be the catalyst that gets the dominos to begin falling. Realize that some people are so emotionally or spiritually paralyzed that they find it nearly impossible to move forward. If you find yourself "stuck" in a rut, I encourage you to take the first step.

For those conducting prayer or prayer ministry:

You will find that praying with scripture in this method may be very helpful. Strongholds are barriers (walls) that significantly retard progress. While praying with scripture may not eliminate all barriers, they may be significantly weakened, allowing progress to be made in a shorter amount of time.

For diseases:

An appendix at the back of this book lists strongholds found in people with various diseases. You can use it to guide you as to where to start. If there are several ailments, you will find considerable overlap of scripture topics.

Sending out scripture lists:

You can give friends a list of scripture verses which are specific to their needs and include instructions on how to pray with scripture. This works particularly well via e-mail. The scripture and prayer could be disease specific or for other needs. For instance, if a friend is apprehensive about things unfolding in his or her life, providing scripture verses pertaining to fear and trust would be very appropriate. It will be such a blessing later when you talk to this friend and find out that the situation has improved.

> *This book should be used anytime you are not at peace, or when you need something about your life to change, but it is not meant to replace anything else you are doing in Jesus' name for healing and transformation.*

Essentials

God will not violate our free will. If you have not surrendered all parts of your life to His Word, what you are about to pray probably will have little effect. If you are praying for yourself, you should give God permission to work in your life by His truth and through the work of the Holy Spirit. Similarly, if you are leading someone else in prayer, you should remind them that they need to give permission to allow God's truth and the Holy Spirit to work in their lives.

Asking for change

Ask Jesus to take the truth of His Word to any place in your life, mind, will, heart, etc., where events or beliefs are not in agreement with God's truth. Ask Jesus to rewrite these false areas with the truth of His Word just as spell check corrects misspelled words on your computer word processing software.

Agreement

You must, on an intellectual level at this time, believe that scripture is the truth. If you don't believe this, there will likely be little change. You will see that there is the topic "Blinded to the Truth of the Word." If you are having trouble reading scripture and understanding it, or your world view doesn't allow you to see the truth, then that topic may be a good place to start.

Praying with scripture may not be the end-all answer, but it certainly can be a significant part of the process of healing and restoration. People who were emotionally wounded as children will need to address those areas. If you are harboring bitterness from unforgiveness, praying with scripture alone may not be enough—you will need to forgive the person to rid yourself of that bitterness. It is mandatory that we forgive in order to get rid of anger and bitterness.

> *God will not violate our free will.*

Praying with these scripture verses will work on negative strongholds such as fear. These strongholds may have developed out of wounds or unforgiven sin, but now have become strongholds in their own right and can stand in the way of healing. Strongholds also can develop out of generational iniquity in your life. Remember the saying "you're a chip off the old block." Traits of past generations carry forward, both good and bad.

Praying for yourself

1. Say the following prayer:

"Heavenly Father, in the name of Jesus, I ask that the scripture verses I read will be accepted as prayer for my life. I further request that you search my entire life, including my heart, soul, and mind, including all memories, to see if there is any conflict with your truth. In addition, I ask that you replace any lies, distortions, or perceptions with the truth of these scriptures."

2. Read the scripture verses you have selected.

Praying for someone else

1. Ask the person if they will allow Jesus to go anywhere in their life to search for conflict, error, lies, or unbelief with the truth of the scripture.

2. Ask if they will allow Jesus to replace any conflict, error, lie, or unbelief with the truth of the scripture.

3. Then pray: "Heavenly Father, in the name of Jesus, I ask that you will search (name)'s entire life, including their heart, soul, and mind, and all memories to see if there is any conflict, error, lie, or unbelief with your truth. Father, I ask if there are any errors, lies, distortions, or misperceptions with the scripture that I read, I pray that these errors will be replaced with the truth of these scripture verses so that everything in (name)'s life conforms to the truth of Your Word."

4. Go through selected scripture verses.

Praying over Children with Scripture

Give Jesus permission to bring truth and healing to your child. Request that the Holy Spirit direct the scripture to where it needs to go: the mind, spirit, soul, and heart. Ask that error and lies be replaced or overwritten with the truth of the scripture. Ask that your child would experientially know and live these truths. Read the scripture verses you have chosen. You may emphasize certain aspects, if you like. For example, Ephesians 2:10 states we are magnificently made, so you might request that Jesus makes sure your child will know that he was magnificently made after reading Ephesians 2:10.

> *Give Jesus permission to bring truth and healing to your child.*

Psychiatrist Dr. Thomas Verny wrote a book *The Secret Life of the Unborn Child* in early 1981. In his practice, he became intrigued about why some children thrive and others don't immediately after birth. He compiled research throughout Europe and North America. Based on scientific medical research, he wrote that unborn babies could be conditioned to a learned behavior. It was found that long-term anxiety (fear) could become a stronghold of fear in unborn babies. This would lead to future problems.

It was further found that when people and animals are in a state of fear they produce a chemical called catecholamine, which circulates in the bloodstream. This chemical will pass through the placenta and the baby will have a physiological fear reaction. So fear can be passed from mother to baby. Depending on the frequency and substance of the fear, the child could be born with gastrointestinal problems. The symptoms sound a little like colic.

Let's look at another scenario. Let's say you are a new grandmother and you visit the mother and child several months after the birth. They are home and have established a routine. Of course, you are dying to hold the baby, and as soon as the mother hands the baby over to you, the baby begins to scream. This situation occurs during subsequent visits. Ah, separation anxiety—or is it? Could it be some conditioned fear, like fear of man? Anxiety is fear.

Another area of consideration is generational iniquity. Praying with these scripture verses over a period of time as a blanket covering makes sense.

Prayer for babies

1. Say the following prayer:

"Heavenly Father, in the name of Jesus I ask that the scripture I read will be accepted as a prayer for (baby's name). I further request that you search (baby's name) entire short life, including his/her heart, soul, and brain, including all memories or strongholds, to see if there is any conflict with your truth. Father, I ask that you replace any lies, distortions, misperceptions, or strongholds with the truth from these scripture verses."

2. Begin to read the scripture verses you selected.

Prayer for children who have some understanding

1. Ask the child if it is okay to read to them. Then ask them if they will allow God to work in their life. You may want to keep this in a more conversational tone if the child is not used to being prayed for.

2. Pray as your would for babies.

3. Go through selected scripture verses.

Accepting God God's Love, and God's Presence

For many of us, having God's presence in our life is a desire that seems just beyond our reach. Others may not even know this desire, but are acquainted with an empty feeling, oftentimes described as "something missing in my life," or there may be an insatiable longing for something unknown. People search for a way to fill that void by pursuing money, power, sex, drugs, religion, materialism, and more, only to find less peace and a greater sense of unfulfillment.

It is in God's presence that we find protection and our needs being met.

> **Psalms 91:1-2** *1 He that dwelleth in the secret place of the Most High Shall abide under the shadow of the Almighty. 2 I will say of Jehovah, He is my refuge and my fortress; My God, in whom I trust.*

In God's presence we learn who God is and what He desires for us. We learn to live in obedience and to start trusting Him. Fear diminishes, thus allowing us to have greater faith in Him and to better follow His will even when faced with various temptations.

Being in God's presence brings us many blessings, such as the fruits of the Spirit listed in Galatians:

> **Galatians 5:22-23** *22 But the fruit of the Spirit is love, joy, peace, longsuffering, kindness, goodness, faithfulness, 23 meekness, self-control; against such there is no law.*

Yet for many, experiencing God's presence is illusive. Why? There are surely many possibilities, but consider this as one: Many know that God is the all-powerful Creator of the universe, and so they assume that God must be to blame when bad things happen.

> *It is in God's presence that we find protection and our needs being met.*

These are common questions that arise:

- Why did He allow bad things to happen in my life?
- Why didn't He protect me?
- Why weren't my needs met?

Several higher concepts about the nature and character of God may help answer these questions.

First, God gave us free will so that we could freely choose to have a relationship and worship Him. If He interferes with our freewill when evil is done, He would also be interfering with our choice to seek Him.

Second, God is impartial and gives everyone equal consideration. Consider the following from Romans and Acts:

> **Romans 2:11** *"For there is no respect of persons with God."*

> **Acts 10:34** *"Peter opened his mouth and said, 'Of a truth I perceive that God is no respecter of persons ...'"*

In other words, God is fair and just. He will respond to people based upon their acknowledgment of Him and the truth that is already in their lives. (See Proverbs 1:24-33.)

For example, as stated in Revelation:

> **Revelation 3:20** *Behold, I stand at the door and knock: if any man hear my voice and open the door, I will come in to him, and will sup with him, and he with me.*

Jesus is at our door quietly knocking, wanting us to let Him in, but He won't come in without an invitation from us.

Third, there are many "if /then" passages in the Bible. Over 1,400 conditional statements are found in scripture, such as "If you follow my commands, then ..." We tend to focus on the "then" verses (the promises) and overlook the "if" verses (our responsibility). We have free will to do as we please, but God is clear that if we don't do it His way, He won't protect us from the consequences.

Fourth, God wants us to utilize our faith. Actions of faith are pleasing to God, and having faith in God is how our Christian life should be lived.

> **Hebrews 11:6** *And without faith it is impossible to be well-pleasing unto him; for he that cometh to God must believe that he is, and that he is a rewarder of them that seek after him.*

Two examples of faith in action are clearly seen in the centurion's conversation with Jesus in Matthew 8:5-13, and in the actions of the friends of the man who was sick with palsy as recorded in Matthew 9:2-7.

Matthew 8:5-13

5 And when he was entered into Capernaum, there came unto him a centurion, beseeching him,

6 and saying, Lord, my servant lieth in the house sick of the palsy, grievously tormented.

7 And he saith unto him, I will come and heal him.

8 And the centurion answered and said, Lord, I am not worthy that thou shouldest come under my roof; but only say the word, and my servant shall be healed.

9 For I also am a man under authority, having under myself soldiers: and I say to this one, Go, and he goeth; and to another, Come, and he cometh; and to my servant, Do this, and he doeth it.

10 And when Jesus heard it, he marvelled, and said to them that followed, Verily I say unto you, I have not found so great faith, no, not in Israel.

11 And I say unto you, that many shall come from the east and the west, and shall sit down with Abraham, and Isaac, and Jacob, in the kingdom of heaven:

12 but the sons of the kingdom shall be cast forth into the outer darkness: there shall be the weeping and the gnashing of teeth.

13 And Jesus said unto the centurion, Go thy way; as thou hast believed, so be it done unto thee. And the servant was healed in that hour.

Matthew 9:2-7

2 And behold, they brought to him a man sick of the palsy, lying on a bed: and Jesus seeing their faith said unto the sick of the palsy, Son, be of good cheer; thy sins are forgiven.

3 And behold, certain of the scribes said within themselves, This man blasphemeth.

4 And Jesus knowing their thoughts said, Wherefore think ye evil in your hearts?

5 For which is easier, to say, Thy sins are forgiven; or to say, Arise, and walk?

6 But that ye may know that the Son of man hath authority on earth to forgive sins (then saith he to the sick of the palsy), Arise, and take

up thy bed, and go up unto thy house.
7 And he arose, and departed to his house.

Joshua reveals an "if/then" word from God:

Joshua 1:6-9

5 There shall not any man be able to stand before thee all the days of thy life. as I was with Moses, so I will be with thee; I will not fail thee, nor forsake thee.
6 Be strong and of good courage; for thou shalt cause this people to inherit the land which I sware unto their fathers to give them.
7 Only be strong and very courageous, to observe to do according to all the law, which Moses my servant commanded thee: turn not from it to the right hand or to the left, that thou mayest have good success whithersoever thou goest.
8 This book of the law shall not depart out of thy mouth, but thou shalt meditate thereon day and night, that thou mayest observe to do according to all that is written therein: for then thou shalt make thy way prosperous, and then thou shalt have good success.
9 Have not I commanded thee? Be strong and of good courage; be not affrighted, neither be thou dismayed: for Jehovah thy God is with thee whithersoever thou goest.

The following passage illustrates that when God works through people, we must act in faith and obedience before something happens.

Joshua 3:15-16

15 and when they that bare the ark were come unto the Jordan, and the feet of the priests that bare the ark were dipped in the brink of the water (for the Jordan overfloweth all its banks all the time of harvest,) 16 that the waters which came down from above stood, and rose up in one heap, a great way off, at Adam, the city that is beside Zarethan; and those that went down toward the sea of the Arabah, even the Salt Sea, were wholly cut off: and the people passed over right against Jericho.

Note that the river didn't part until the feet of the priest went into the water. They acted first in faith. The lesson here is that we need to act in faith. If we hop from church to church hoping God will show up and fix what we incorrectly blamed on Him as being responsible for, we will be very disappointed.

Fifth, when evil occurs, we will immediately blame the perpetrators. But there can also be a transference of blame to God if we are not careful. If we don't correctly answer such questions as "why didn't He protect me?" and "why did He let this happen?" the blame can be transferred to God. Then God can also become our object of unresolved anger. Anger festers and expands into bitterness. The only antidote for bitterness is forgiveness. In essence, we construct a barrier, or wall, that blocks out God's presence in our lives.

> *God can become our object of unresolved anger. We block out God's presence in our lives.*

Sixth, if we blame God for our situation, we expect Him to fix it, and we wait for Him to do it. Some of us might even hop from one church to another hoping He might show up. Many people stick their toe into the spiritual water but go no further because their pride tells them that God broke it, so it's up to Him to fix it. Then, we allow our trust in God to diminish if our situation is not remedied: God can't be relied on. So we don't trust Him or think of sharing our most personal thoughts with Him, which is ironic since He knows everything anyway.

This means if we want to live in God's presence, we must act on it. If we have a barrier of unforgiveness, we must initiate forgiveness toward God. If we don't love God, then receiving love, loving ourself, or loving our neighbor may be difficult. The great news is that we can ask the Holy Spirit to help us with all of this. There may be barriers such as fear, pride, unbelief, or other strongholds that you will need to address. In fact, most of the categories in this book are applicable to barriers that may be in our life that block God's presence, and hence are barriers to receiving God's blessings.

So, if you know that you, or someone else you are helping, has a barrier between themself and God, you will need to visit several scripture topics for sure. How can you tell if this barrier exists? If you or they answer "yes" to either of the following questions, there is likely a barrier.

- Are there questions concerning God's action or lack of help?
- Is there resistance in asking God to help or taking the next step in spiritual growth?

You can start by working on these suggested scripture topics: Anger, Blinded by the Truth of the Word, Faith, Forgiveness, Obedience, Pride, and Trust.

Psalms 5:10
Hold them guilty, O God; Let them fall by their own counsels; Thrust them out in the multitude of their transgressions; For they have rebelled against thee.

Let God help you see what is in the way.

Remember!
When praying scripture, give Jesus permission to search for lies and unbelief and replace them with God's truth.

Revelation 3:20   Key Verse
20 Behold, I stand at the door and knock: if any man hear my voice and open the door, I will come in to him, and will sup with him, and he with me.

Hebrews 9:24   Key Verse
24 For Christ entered not into a holy place made with hands, like in pattern to the true; but into heaven itself, now to appear before the face of God for us:

Hebrews 10:36
36 For ye have need of patience, that, having done the will of God, ye may receive the promise.

1 Kings 8:59
59 And let these my words, wherewith I have made supplication before Jehovah, be nigh unto Jehovah our God day and night, that he maintain the cause of his servant, and the cause of his people Israel, as every day shall require;

Psalms 27:4
4 One thing have I asked of Jehovah, that will I seek after; That I may dwell in the house of Jehovah all the days of my life, To behold the beauty of Jehovah, And to inquire in his temple.

Psalms 61:7
7 He shall abide before God for ever: Oh prepare lovingkindness and truth, that they may preserve him.

Psalms 91:1

1 He that dwelleth in the secret place of the Most High Shall abide under the shadow of the Almighty.

Psalms 100:3

3 Know ye that Jehovah, he is God: It is he that hath made us, and we are his; We are his people, and the sheep of his pasture.

Isaiah 4:5

5 And Jehovah will create over the whole habitation of mount Zion, and over her assemblies, a cloud and smoke by day, and the shining of a flaming fire by night; for over all the glory shall be spread a covering.

Mark 12:24

24 Jesus said unto them, Is it not for this cause that ye err, that ye know not the scriptures, nor the power of God?

Luke 9:11

11 But the multitudes perceiving it followed him: and he welcomed them, and spake to them of the kingdom of God, and them that had need of healing he cured.

John 14:21-24

21 He that hath my commandments, and keepeth them, he it is that loveth me: and he that loveth me shall be loved of my Father, and I will love him, and will manifest myself unto him.
22 Judas (not Iscariot) saith unto him, Lord, what is come to pass that thou wilt manifest thyself unto us, and not unto the world?
23 Jesus answered and said unto him, If a man love me, he will keep my word: and my Father will love him, and we will come unto him, and make our abode with him.
24 He that loveth me not keepeth not my words: and the word which ye hear is not mine, but the Father's who sent me.

John 14:31

31 but that the world may know that I love the Father, and as the Father gave me commandment, even so I do. Arise, let us go hence.

Acts 26:22-23

22 Having therefore obtained the help that is from God, I stand unto this day testifying both to small and great, saying nothing but what the prophets and Moses did say should come;
23 how that the Christ must suffer, and how that he first by the resurrection of the dead should proclaim light both to the people and to the Gentiles.

Romans 13:2

2 Therefore he that resisteth the power, withstandeth the ordinance of God: and they that withstand shall receive to themselves judgment.

1 Corinthians 3:16

16 Know ye not that ye are a temple of God, and that the Spirit of God dwelleth in you?

1 Corinthians 12:24

24 whereas our comely parts have no need: but God tempered the body together, giving more abundant honor to that part which lacked;

Philippians 4:6

6 In nothing be anxious; but in everything by prayer and supplication with thanksgiving let your requests be made known unto God.

Philippians 4:19

19 And my God shall supply every need of yours according to his riches in glory in Christ Jesus.

Titus 1:16

16 They profess that they know God; but by their works they deny him, being abominable, and disobedient, and unto every good work reprobate.

1 John 3:17

17 But whoso hath the world's goods, and beholdeth his brother in need, and shutteth up his compassion from him, how doth the love of God abide in him?

2 John 1:6

6 And this is love, that we should walk after his commandments. This is the commandment, even as ye heard from the beginning, that ye should walk in it.

Jude 1:4

4 For there are certain men crept in privily, even they who were of old written of beforehand unto this condemnation, ungodly men, turning the grace of our God into lasciviousness, and denying our only Master and Lord, Jesus Christ.

Accepting the Trustworthiness of God's Word

Jesus is the center of our faith. God's written Word is our foundation for developing knowledge and belief. If you don't trust God's Word, how can you move forward in faith? How can you tap into the power of His Word? Will scripture be able to help you remove strongholds if you don't trust God's Word? If you aren't fully certain that you can trust scripture, then you may need to pray with these scripture verses.

Remember!
When praying scripture, give Jesus permission to search for lies and unbelief and replace them with God's truth.

Isaiah 55:11 Key Verse
11 so shall my word be that goeth forth out of my mouth: it shall not return unto me void, but it shall accomplish that which I please, and it shall prosper in the thing whereto I sent it.

2 Timothy 3:16   Key Verse
16 Every scripture inspired of God is also profitable for teaching, for reproof, for correction, for instruction which is in righteousness.

Luke 21:33   Key Verse
33 Heaven and earth shall pass away: but my words shall not pass away.

Numbers 23:19
19 God is not a man, that he should lie, Neither the son of man, that he should repent: Hath he said, and will he not do it? Or hath he spoken, and will he not make it good?

Joshua 1:8
8 This book of the law shall not depart out of thy mouth, but thou shalt meditate thereon day and night, that thou mayest observe to do according to all that is written therein: for then thou shalt make thy way prosperous, and then thou shalt have good success.

Psalms 18:30
30 As for God, his way is perfect: The word of Jehovah is tried; He is a shield unto all them that take refuge in him.

Psalms 30:5
5 For his anger is but for a moment; His favor is for a life-time: Weeping may tarry for the night, But joy cometh in the morning.

Psalms 56:4
4 In God (I will praise his word), In God have I put my trust, I will not be afraid; What can flesh do unto me?

Psalms 119:11
11 Thy word have I laid up in my heart, That I might not sin against thee.

Psalms 119:42

42 So shall I have an answer for him that reproacheth me; For I trust in thy word.

Psalms 119:89

89 For ever, O Jehovah, Thy word is settled in heaven.

Jeremiah 1:12

12 Then said Jehovah unto me, Thou hast well seen: for I watch over my word to perform it.

Mark 13:31

31 Heaven and earth shall pass away: but my words shall not pass away.

Hebrews 4:12

12 For the word of God is living, and active, and sharper than any two-edged sword, and piercing even to the dividing of soul and spirit, of both joints and marrow, and quick to discern the thoughts and intents of the heart.

Hebrews 10:16

16 This is the covenant that I will make with them. After those days, saith the Lord: I will put my laws on their heart, And upon their mind also will I write them; then saith he …

1 Peter 1:25

25 But the word of the Lord abideth for ever. And this is the word of good tidings which was preached unto you.

Anger, Bitterness, Hate, Resentment, and Murder

This topic includes self-anger, self-hate, etc. "Self" is used to describe the emotion when it is directed at one's self.

Anger is a very destructive emotion, but it is an emotion that God gave us. It is not wrong to get angry. Even Jesus got angry, as evidenced when He turned the money tables over in the temple. However, Jesus exhibited righteous anger—He did not act upon His anger to commit sin. Scripture is clear that our anger moves us into sin if we don't let it go before the end of the day.

Anger can be something we take ownership of because it can be a cornerstone of who we believe we are. It could be the only thing a person may believe he truly owns outright. The problem is, we act out on anger in ways that are destructive to relationships, and this will lead to regrettable consequences. Like a hurricane that increases in stages, anger can develop into bitterness, hate, rage, and murder.

For some of us, anger may not be obvious; it may be imbedded in a memory of our past. This anger may stop us from wanting the freeing release provided by forgiveness because we savor the feeling of anger or we use angry outbursts to control people. When anger turns into bitterness, it will eat at our soul like cancer eats at our flesh. Even medical science sees this connection.

Anger can be self-directed. People have been known to cut themselves, showing they have progressed to self-hate. The link at the end of that chain is murder—in the form of suicide!

There appears to be a connection between rebellion and anger. If a person has been hurt by someone, anger may fester from an incident if it is not forgiven. If there do not appear to be any consequences for the offender, the victim may become rebellious, find injustice and unfairness everywhere, and take offense at everything. The rebellion creates a big divide between the once victim and God, all sorts of other people, and even society in general.

> *The problem is, we act out on anger in ways that are destructive to relationships, and this will lead to regrettable consequences.*

We have control over the forgiveness, but must trust and leave the justice part to God. Read Psalm 58 and pray with it, if appropriate, just like David did.

Remember!
When praying scripture, give Jesus permission to search for lies and unbelief and replace them with God's truth.

Ephesians 4:31-32 Key Verse
31 Let all bitterness, and wrath, and anger, and clamor, and railing, be put away from you, with all malice:
32 and be ye kind one to another, tenderhearted, forgiving each other, even as God also in Christ forgave you.

Ephesians 4:26-27   Key Verse
26 Be ye angry, and sin not: let not the sun go down upon your wrath:
27 neither give place to the devil.

Hebrews 12:15   Key Verse
15 looking carefully lest there be any man that falleth short of the grace of God; lest any root of bitterness springing up trouble you, and thereby the many be defiled;

Leviticus 26:28
28 then I will walk contrary unto you in wrath; and I also will chastise you seven times for your sins.

Deuteronomy 29:19
19 and it come to pass, when he heareth the words of this curse, that he bless himself in his heart, saying, I shall have peace, though I walk in the stubbornness of my heart, to destroy the moist with the dry.

Deuteronomy 32:32
32 For their vine is of the vine of Sodom, And of the fields of Gomorrah: Their grapes are grapes of gall, Their clusters are bitter...

Job 5:2
2 For vexation killeth the foolish man, And jealousy slayeth the silly one

Job 36:13
13 But they that are godless in heart lay up anger: They cry not for help when he bindeth them.

Job 40:11
11 Pour forth the overflowings of thine anger; And look upon every one that is proud, and abase him.

Proverbs 6:34
34 For jealousy is the rage of a man; And he will not spare in the day of vengeance.

Proverbs 25:21-22
21 If thine enemy be hungry, give him bread to eat; And if he be thirsty, give him water to drink:
22 For thou wilt heap coals of fire upon his head, And Jehovah will reward thee.

Proverbs 29:9
9 If a wise man hath a controversy with a foolish man, Whether he be angry or laugh, there will be no rest.

Isaiah 37:29
29 Because of thy raging against me, and because thine arrogancy is come up into mine ears, therefore will I put my hook in thy nose, and my bridle in thy lips, and I will turn thee back by the way by which thou camest

Jeremiah 4:18
18 Thy way and thy doings have procured these things unto thee; this is thy wickedness; for it is bitter, for it reacheth unto thy heart.

Hosea 7:16
16 They return, but not to him that is on high; they are like a deceitful bow; their princes shall fall by the sword for the rage of their tongue: this shall be their derision in the land of Egypt.

Matthew 5:22
22 but I say unto you, that every one who is angry with his brother shall be in danger of the judgment; and whosoever shall say to his brother, Raca, shall be in danger of the council; and whosoever shall say, Thou fool, shall be in danger of the hell of fire.

Mark 7:21

21 For from within, out of the heart of men, evil thoughts proceed, fornications, thefts, murders, adulteries,

Acts 8:23

23 For I see that thou art in the gall of bitterness and in the bond of iniquity.

Romans 12:19-21

19 Avenge not yourselves, beloved, but give place unto the wrath of God: for it is written, Vengeance belongeth unto me; I will recompense, saith the Lord.
20 But if thine enemy hunger, feed him; if he thirst, give him to drink: for in so doing thou shalt heap coals of fire upon his head.
21 Be not overcome of evil, but overcome evil with good.

Colossians 3:8

8 but now do ye also put them all away: anger, wrath, malice, railing, shameful speaking out of your mouth:

James 3:4

4 Behold, the ships also, though they are so great and are driven by rough winds, are yet turned about by a very small rudder, whither the impulse of the steersman willeth.

BLINDED TO THE TRUTH OF THE WORD

Are you unable to concentrate when reading the Bible? Does it not make sense? You may have an obstacle that's stopping you from understanding, or there may be other obstacles, such as fear and your identity. But allowing God to touch some of your blind spots with His Word may be just what you need to get you started on the right path. Allow the Word, guided by the Holy Spirit, to bring light into the dark areas of your heart.

 Remember!
When praying scripture, give Jesus permission to search for lies and unbelief and replace them with God's truth.

John 12:40 Key Verse
40 He hath blinded their eyes, and he hardened their heart; Lest they should see with their eyes, and perceive with their heart, And should turn, And I should heal them.

Mark 4:9   Key Verse
9 And he said, Who hath ears to hear, let him hear.

Ephesians 4:18-19   Key Verse
18 being darkened in their understanding, alienated from the life of God, because of the ignorance that is in them, because of the hardening of their heart;
19 who being past feeling gave themselves up to lasciviousness, to work all uncleanness with greediness.

Psalms 95:10   Key Verse
10 Forty years long was I grieved with that generation, And said, It is a people that do err in their heart, And they have not known my ways:

1 Samuel 3:9
9 Therefore Eli said unto Samuel, Go, lie down: and it shall be, if he call thee, that thou shalt say, Speak, Jehovah; for thy servant heareth. So Samuel went and lay down in his place.

2 Kings 6:16-17
16 And he answered, Fear not; for they that are with us are more than they that are with them.
17 And Elisha prayed, and said, Jehovah, I pray thee, open his eyes, that he may see. And Jehovah opened the eyes of the young man; and he saw: and, behold, the mountain was full of horses and chariots of fire round about Elisha.

2 Chronicles 7:14
14 if my people, who are called by my name, shall humble themselves, and pray, and seek my face, and turn from their wicked ways; then will I hear from heaven, and will forgive their sin, and will heal their land.

Job 15:31
31 Let him not trust in vanity, deceiving himself; For vanity shall be

his recompense.

Psalms 18:28
28 For thou wilt light my lamp: Jehovah my God will lighten my darkness.

Psalms 119:144
144 Thy testimonies are righteous for ever: Give me understanding, and I shall live.

Psalms 139:11-12
11 If I say, Surely the darkness shall overwhelm me, And the light about me shall be night;
12 Even the darkness hideth not from thee, But the night shineth as the day: The darkness and the light are both alike to thee.

Proverbs 16:20
20 He that giveth heed unto the word shall find good; And whoso trusteth in Jehovah, happy is he.

Isaiah 5:13
13 Therefore my people are gone into captivity for lack of knowledge; and their honorable men are famished, and their multitude are parched with thirst.

Isaiah 42:16
16 And I will bring the blind by a way that they know not; in paths that they know not will I lead them; I will make darkness light before them, and crooked places straight. These things will I do, and I will not forsake them.

Jeremiah 4:22
22 For my people are foolish, they know me not; they are sottish children, and they have no understanding; they are wise to do evil, but to do good they have no knowledge.

Jeremiah 6:10
10 To whom shall I speak and testify, that they may hear? behold, their ear is uncircumcised, and they cannot hearken: behold, the word of Jehovah is become unto them a reproach; they have no delight in it.

Jeremiah 7:22-24
22 For I spake not unto your fathers, nor commanded them in the day that I brought them out of the land of Egypt, concerning burnt-offerings or sacrifices:
23 but this thing I commanded them, saying, Hearken unto my voice, and I will be your God, and ye shall be my people; and walk ye in all the way that I command you, that it may be well with you.
24 But they hearkened not, nor inclined their ear, but walked in their own counsels and in the stubbornness of their evil heart, and went backward, and not forward.

Ezekiel 12:2
2 Son of man, thou dwellest in the midst of the rebellious house, that have eyes to see, and see not, that have ears to hear, and hear not; for they are a rebellious house.

Zechariah 7:11
11 But they refused to hearken, and pulled away the shoulder, and stopped their ears, that they might not hear.

Matthew 4:4
4 But he answered and said, It is written, Man shall not live by bread alone, but by every word that proceedeth out of the mouth of God.

Matthew 4:16
16 the people that sat in darkness saw a great light, and to them that sat in the region and shadow of death, to them did light spring up.

Matthew 11:5

5 the blind receive their sight, and the lame walk, the lepers are cleansed, and the deaf hear, and the dead are raised up, and the poor have good tidings preached to them.

Matthew 13:15

15 For this people's heart is waxed gross, And their ears are dull of hearing, And their eyes they have closed; Lest haply they should perceive with their eyes, And hear with their ears, And understand with their heart, And should turn again, And I should heal them.

Mark 4:22-24

22 For there is nothing hid, save that it should be manifested; neither was anything made secret, but that it should come to light.
23 If any man hath ears to hear, let him hear.
24 And he said unto them, Take heed what ye hear: with what measure ye mete it shall be measured unto you; and more shall be given unto you.

Luke 11:28

28 But he said, Yea rather, blessed are they that hear the word of God, and keep it.

John 1:5

5 And the light shineth in the darkness; and the darkness apprehended it not.

John 8:12

12 Again therefore Jesus spake unto them, saying, I am the light of the world: he that followeth me shall not walk in the darkness, but shall have the light of life.

John 9:39-41

39 And Jesus said, For judgment came I into this world, that they that see not may see; and that they that see may become blind.
40 Those of the Pharisees who were with him heard these things,

and said unto him, Are we also blind?
41 Jesus said unto them, If ye were blind, ye would have no sin: but now ye say, We see: your sin remaineth.

John 10:10
10 The thief cometh not, but that he may steal, and kill, and destroy: I came that they may have life, and may have it abundantly.

John 16:16
16 A little while, and ye behold me no more; and again a little while, and ye shall see me.

John 17:17
17 Sanctify them in the truth: thy word is truth.

Acts 28:26
26 saying, Go thou unto this people, and say, By hearing ye shall hear, and shall in no wise understand; And seeing ye shall see, and shall in no wise perceive:

Romans 6:23
23 For the wages of sin is death; but the free gift of God is eternal life in Christ Jesus our Lord.

1 Corinthians 2:10-12
10 But unto us God revealed them through the Spirit: for the Spirit searcheth all things, yea, the deep things of God.
11 For who among men knoweth the things of a man, save the spirit of the man, which is in him? even so the things of God none knoweth, save the Spirit of God.
12 But we received, not the spirit of the world, but the spirit which is from God; that we might know the things that were freely given to us of God.

2 Corinthians 4:3-6
3 And even if our gospel is veiled, it is veiled in them that perish:

4 in whom the god of this world hath blinded the minds of the unbelieving, that the light of the gospel of the glory of Christ, who is the image of God, should not dawn upon them.
5 For we preach not ourselves, but Christ Jesus as Lord, and ourselves as your servants for Jesus' sake.
6 Seeing it is God, that said, Light shall shine out of darkness, who shined in our hearts, to give the light of the knowledge of the glory of God in the face of Jesus Christ.

2 Corinthians 11:3
3 But I fear, lest by any means, as the serpent beguiled Eve in his craftiness, your minds should be corrupted from the simplicity and the purity that is toward Christ.

Ephesians 1:15-23 (Paul's prayer for spiritual wisdom)
15 For this cause I also, having heard of the faith in the Lord Jesus which is among you, and the love which ye show toward all the saints,
16 cease not to give thanks for you, making mention of you in my prayers;
17 that the God of our Lord Jesus Christ, the Father of glory, may give unto you a spirit of wisdom and revelation in the knowledge of him;
18 having the eyes of your heart enlightened, that ye may know what is the hope of his calling, what the riches of the glory of his inheritance in the saints,
19 and what the exceeding greatness of his power to us-ward who believe, according to that working of the strength of his might
20 which he wrought in Christ, when he raised him from the dead, and made him to sit at his right hand in the heavenly places,
21 far above all rule, and authority, and power, and dominion, and every name that is named, not only in this world, but also in that which is to come:
22 and he put all things in subjection under his feet, and gave him to be head over all things to the church,
23 which is his body, the fulness of him that filleth all in all.

Ephesians 2:2

2 wherein ye once walked according to the course of this world, according to the prince of the powers of the air, of the spirit that now worketh in the sons of disobedience;

Colossians 1:15-17

15 who is the image of the invisible God, the firstborn of all creation;

16 for in him were all things created, in the heavens and upon the earth, things visible and things invisible, whether thrones or dominions or principalities or powers; all things have been created through him, and unto him;

17 and he is before all things, and in him all things consist.

Colossians 2:8

8 Take heed lest there shall be any one that maketh spoil of you through his philosophy and vain deceit, after the tradition of men, after the rudiments of the world, and not after Christ:

Colossians 3:16

16 Let the word of Christ dwell in you richly; in all wisdom teaching and admonishing one another with psalms and hymns and spiritual songs, singing with grace in your hearts unto God.

1 Timothy 1:6-7

6 from which things some having swerved have turned aside unto vain talking;

7 desiring to be teachers of the law, though they understand neither what they say, nor whereof they confidently affirm.

2 Timothy 2:25-26

25 in meekness correcting them that oppose themselves; if peradventure God may give them repentance unto the knowledge of the truth,

26 and they may recover themselves out of the snare of the devil, having been taken captive by him unto his will.

2 Timothy 4:4
4 and will turn away their ears from the truth, and turn aside unto fables.

Hebrews 4:2
2 For indeed we have had good tidings preached unto us, even as also they: but the word of hearing did not profit them, because it was not united by faith with them that heard.

Hebrews 4:11
11 Let us therefore give diligence to enter into that rest, that no man fall after the same example of disobedience.

James 1:5-8
5 But if any of you lacketh wisdom, let him ask of God, who giveth to all liberally and upbraideth not; and it shall be given him.
6 But let him ask in faith, nothing doubting: for he that doubteth is like the surge of the sea driven by the wind and tossed.
7 For let not that man think that he shall receive anything of the Lord;
8 a doubleminded man, unstable in all his ways.

James 1:22
22 But be ye doers of the word, and not hearers only, deluding your own selves.

1 John 1:5
5 And this is the message which we have heard from him and announce unto you, that God is light, and in him is no darkness at all.

Character of God

Man was made in the image of God. Genesis 1:27 states: *"And God created man in his own image, in the image of God created he him; male and female created he them."* How we view God reflects how we view ourselves. Our dignity and self-worth will be affected by these beliefs. Viewing God as harsh will cause us to understand our position in Christ differently than viewing God as loving.

> **A harsh view of God may result in a very condemning opinion of ourselves.**

A harsh view of God may result in a very condemning opinion of ourselves. Taking a legalistic view can make it difficult to accept God's grace. These feelings harden our heart, which further separates us from God.

Those who have a strict, critical, and controlling father may subconsciously transfer these attributes onto Father God. Certain biblical teachings may also contribute to our view of God. Jesus said that He came to earth to show us the nature of His Father. Love, grace, mercy, and forgiveness are some of the attributes we see in Jesus, which we should realize are part of the nature and character of Father God.

Because we base our self-value on what we believe God thinks of us, we must know His true nature. Otherwise we will have a distorted view of ourselves, which can result in all sorts of self-destructive thinking and actions. If you have a difficult time believing in your salvation, then knowing God's character may help greatly.

> **Remember!**
> When praying scripture, give Jesus permission to search for lies and unbelief and replace them with God's truth.

Exodus 34:6   Key Verse
6 And Jehovah passed by before him, and proclaimed, Jehovah, Jehovah, a God merciful and gracious, slow to anger, and abundant in lovingkindness and truth,

Psalms 33:5   Key Verse
5 He loveth righteousness and justice: The earth is full of the lovingkindness of Jehovah.

Deuteronomy 32:4   Key Verse
4 The Rock, his work is perfect; For all his ways are justice: A God of faithfulness and without iniquity, Just and right is he.

Genesis 1:27
27 And God created man in his own image, in the image of God created he him; male and female created he them.

Exodus 18:9
9 And Jethro rejoiced for all the goodness which Jehovah had done

to Israel, in that he had delivered them out of the hand of the Egyptians.

1 Chronicles 16:34
34 O give thanks unto Jehovah; for he is good; For his lovingkindness endureth for ever.

Psalms 18:30
30 As for God, his way is perfect: The word of Jehovah is tried; He is a shield unto all them that take refuge in him.

Psalms 25:8
8 Good and upright is Jehovah: Therefore will he instruct sinners in the way.

Psalms 36:5
5 Thy lovingkindness, O Jehovah, is in the heavens; Thy faithfulness reacheth unto the skies.

Psalms 86:5
5 For thou, Lord, art good, and ready to forgive, And abundant in lovingkindness unto all them that call upon thee.

Psalms 100:5
5 For Jehovah is good; His lovingkindness endureth for ever, And his faithfulness unto all generations.

Joel 2:13
13 and rend your heart, and not your garments, and turn unto Jehovah your God; for he is gracious and merciful, slow to anger, and abundant in lovingkindness, and repenteth him of the evil.

John 3:16
16 For God so loved the world, that he gave his only begotten Son, that whosoever believeth on him should not perish, but have eternal life.

Romans 4:21
21 and being fully assured that what he had promised, he was able also to perform.

Romans 8:32
32 He that spared not his own Son, but delivered him up for us all, how shall he not also with him freely give us all things?

Romans 8:38-39
38 For I am persuaded, that neither death, nor life, nor angels, nor principalities, nor things present, nor things to come, nor powers,
39 nor height, nor depth, nor any other creature, shall be able to separate us from the love of God, which is in Christ Jesus our Lord.

Ephesians 2:4-6
4 but God, being rich in mercy, for his great love wherewith he loved us,
5 even when we were dead through our trespasses, made us alive together with Christ (by grace have ye been saved),
6 and raised us up with him, and made us to sit with him in the heavenly places, in Christ Jesus:

Titus 3:5
5 not by works done in righteousness, which we did ourselves, but according to his mercy he saved us, through the washing of regeneration and renewing of the Holy Spirit,

James 1:17
17 Every good gift and every perfect gift is from above, coming down from the Father of lights, with whom can be no variation, neither shadow that is cast by turning.

1 John 3:16
16 Hereby know we love, because he laid down his life for us: and we ought to lay down our lives for the brethren.

1 John 4:7

7 Beloved, let us love one another: for love is of God; and every one that loveth is begotten of God, and knoweth God.

1 John 4:10

10 Herein is love, not that we loved God, but that he loved us, and sent his Son to be the propitiation for our sins.

Comfort, Contentment, Discouragement, Jealousy, and Envy

God is the real source of comfort and contentment, and the best antidote to discouragement. Other sources will let us down. True comfort in the Lord is a state of being which brings confidence and a sense of rest to our inner person. This kind of comfort does not come from having a nice home or other worldly possessions. Contentment means living in peace and joy, no matter what you have. Yet many of us feel discouraged if we have not obtained what we think we should in our lifetime. God will provide, but He decides what and when.

> **Contentment means living in peace and joy, no matter what you have.**

The peace in all of this comes from trusting that it is so. Lack of trust in God makes us vulnerable to trap doors, which will take us down. Consider envy, for example. It can eat at us. According to Proverbs 14:30, *"A tranquil heart is the life of the flesh; But envy is the rottenness of the bones."* This trap door sounds like osteoporosis. Jealousy and envy are signs that we lack comfort and contentment. If jealousy and envy are in us, we cannot have peace at the same time.

When stressed, some people will overeat. Food then becomes a source of comfort. Instead of overeating, as an alternative, look to Jesus for comfort.

If there is a lack of satisfaction in your life, then you could use some of the following verses.

> **Remember!**
> When praying scripture, give Jesus permission to search for lies and unbelief and replace them with God's truth.

2 Thessalonians 2:16-17   Key Verse
16 Now our Lord Jesus Christ himself, and God our Father who loved us and gave us eternal comfort and good hope through grace, 17 comfort your hearts and establish them in every good work and word.

Psalms 55:22   Key Verse
22 Cast thy burden upon Jehovah, and he will sustain thee: He will never suffer the righteous to be moved.

Psalms 42:6-11
6 O my God, my soul is cast down within me: Therefore do I remember thee from the land of the Jordan, And the Hermons, from the hill Mizar.
7 Deep calleth unto deep at the noise of thy waterfalls: All thy waves and thy billows are gone over me.
8 Yet Jehovah will command his lovingkindness in the day-time; And in the night his song shall be with me, Even a prayer unto the

God of my life.
9 I will say unto God my rock, Why hast thou forgotten me? Why go I mourning because of the oppression of the enemy?
10 As with a sword in my bones, mine adversaries reproach me, While they continually say unto me, Where is thy God?
11 Why art thou cast down, O my soul? And why art thou disquieted within me? Hope thou in God; For I shall yet praise him, Who is the help of my countenance, and my God.

Nahum 1:7
7 Jehovah is good, a stronghold in the day of trouble; and he knoweth them that take refuge in him.

Matthew 5:4
4 Blessed are they that mourn: for they shall be comforted.

John 14:16
16 And I will pray the Father, and he shall give you another Comforter, that he may be with you for ever,

2 Corinthians 4:8-9
8 we are pressed on every side, yet not straitened; perplexed, yet not unto despair;
9 pursued, yet not forsaken; smitten down, yet not destroyed;

Galatians 4:6-7
6 And because ye are sons, God sent forth the Spirit of his Son into our hearts, crying, Abba, Father.
7 So that thou art no longer a bondservant, but a son; and if a son, then an heir through God.

Ephesians 4:29
29 Let no corrupt speech proceed out of your mouth, but such as is good for edifying as the need may be, that it may give grace to them that hear.

Philippians 4:12-13

12 I know how to be abased, and I know also how to abound: in everything and in all things have I learned the secret both to be filled and to be hungry, both to abound and to be in want.
13 I can do all things in him that strengtheneth me.

Colossians 2:2

2 that their hearts may be comforted, they being knit together in love, and unto all riches of the full assurance of understanding, that they may know the mystery of God, even Christ,

Discernment

The dictionary defines discern as "to perceive by the sight or some other sense, or by the intellect; see, recognize or differentiate; discriminate." Perhaps you know people who are traveling through life with no idea of what is going on around them. They don't see the big sign—Danger, land mines!—and are walking around with explosions going off around them. Most certainly they will get hurt, as well as those in their charge and those in relationships with them. Life can be dangerous. We teach our children to watch out for danger, such as traffic. These are dangers of the physical world, which we should see.

There are also grave dangers in the spiritual world, the world we do not see. Some people seem to be aware of these dangers even though they cannot see them. We call this "discernment," in a biblical sense. When we become Christians we are given spiritual gifts, and some of us receive these gifts in abundance.

> *There are also grave dangers in the spiritual world, the world we do not see.*

Yet like all of our talents given by God, we must develop them just as a young child must develop the ability to walk.

If you ask God to give you the gift of discernment, He probably will, but it is up to you to develop it. Being able to sense evil around us and dangers on the horizon can do much for our life. There are people and places we should know to stay away from, or at least remain at arm's length if total avoidance is not possible.

Remember!
When praying scripture, give Jesus permission to search for lies and unbelief and replace them with God's truth.

1 John 4:1   Key Verse
1 Beloved, believe not every spirit, but prove the spirits, whether they are of God; because many false prophets are gone out into the world.

Colossians 2:18   Key Verse
18 Let no man rob you of your prize by a voluntary humility and worshipping of the angels, dwelling in the things which he hath seen, vainly puffed up by his fleshly mind,

2 Kings 6:17   Key Verse
17 And Elisha prayed, and said, Jehovah, I pray thee, open his eyes, that he may see. And Jehovah opened the eyes of the young man; and he saw: and, behold, the mountain was full of horses and chariots of fire round about Elisha.

Proverbs 28:5
5 Evil men understand not justice; But they that seek Jehovah understand all things.

Jeremiah 17:9

9 The heart is deceitful above all things, and it is exceedingly corrupt: who can know it?

Matthew 13:24-28

24 Another parable set he before them, saying, The kingdom of heaven is likened unto a man that sowed good seed in his field:
25 but while men slept, his enemy came and sowed tares also among the wheat, and went away.
26 But when the blade sprang up and brought forth fruit, then appeared the tares also.
27 And the servants of the householder came and said unto him, Sir, didst thou not sow good seed in thy field? whence then hath it tares?
28 And he said unto them, An enemy hath done this. And the servants say unto him, Wilt thou then that we go and gather them up?

Matthew 13:30

30 Let both grow together until the harvest: and in the time of the harvest I will say to the reapers, Gather up first the tares, and bind them in bundles to burn them; but gather the wheat into my barn.

Matthew 7:15-17

15 Beware of false prophets, who come to you in sheep's clothing, but inwardly are ravening wolves.
16 By their fruits ye shall know them. Do men gather grapes of thorns, or figs of thistles?
17 Even so every good tree bringeth forth good fruit; but the corrupt tree bringeth forth evil fruit.

Mark 5:30

30 And straightway Jesus, perceiving in himself that the power proceeding from him had gone forth, turned him about in the crowd, and said, Who touched my garments?

1 Corinthians 2:15

15 But he that is spiritual judgeth all things, and he himself is judged of no man.

Ephesians 1:17-18

17 that the God of our Lord Jesus Christ, the Father of glory, may give unto you a spirit of wisdom and revelation in the knowledge of him;

18 having the eyes of your heart enlightened, that ye may know what is the hope of his calling, what the riches of the glory of his inheritance in the saints,

Faith

Faith is the essence of Christianity. Without faith, we are not saved, *"For God so loved the world, that he gave his only begotten Son, that whosoever believeth on him should not perish, but have eternal life* (John 3:16)." Jesus told some, but not all, that they were healed by their faith. Where does faith come from? Romans 12:3 tells us that God has already given us a measure of faith. In the Greek translation, the word for "measure" means ability or capacity. So, God has already given us the ability and capacity for living in faith. Romans 10:17 tells us that our faith can be increased by hearing the Good News—the Word of God! Sometimes just seeing transformed lives—that of our own or others—encourages us and helps to grow our faith.

> **Sometimes just seeing transformed lives encourages us and helps to grow our faith.**

Many want to have a strong belief, but their faith is weak. Knowledge of scripture will help greatly. There is something else you can do about weak faith—pray. Consider Paul's prayer to the Ephesians:

Ephesians 1:15-23
15 For this cause I also, having heard of the faith in the Lord Jesus which is among you, and the love which ye show toward all the saints, 16 cease not to give thanks for you, making mention of you in my prayers; 17 that the God of our Lord Jesus Christ, the Father of glory, may give unto you a spirit of wisdom and revelation in the knowledge of him; 18 having the eyes of your heart enlightened, that ye may know what is the hope of his calling, what the riches of the glory of his inheritance in the saints, 19 and what the exceeding greatness of his power to us-ward who believe, according to that working of the strength of his might 20 which he wrought in Christ, when he raised him from the dead, and made him to sit at his right hand in the heavenly places, 21 far above all rule, and authority, and power, and dominion, and every name that is named, not only in this world, but also in that which is to come: 22 and he put all things in subjection under his feet, and gave him to be head over all things to the church, 23 which is his body, the fulness of him that filleth all in all.

Remember!
When praying scripture, give Jesus permission to search for lies and unbelief and replace them with God's truth.

Matthew 19:26 Key Verse
26 And Jesus looking upon them said to them, With men this is impossible; but with God all things are possible.

Luke 11:9-10 Key Verse
9 And I say unto you, Ask, and it shall be given you; seek, and ye shall find; knock, and it shall be opened unto you.
10 For every one that asketh receiveth; and he that seeketh findeth; and to him that knocketh it shall be opened.

John 20:29 Key Verse
29 Jesus saith unto him, Because thou hast seen me, thou hast believed: blessed are they that have not seen, and yet have believed.

Psalms 27:13
13 I had fainted, unless I had believed to see the goodness of Jehovah In the land of the living.

Matthew 17:20
20 And he saith unto them, Because of your little faith: for verily I say unto you, If ye have faith as a grain of mustard seed, ye shall say unto this mountain, Remove hence to yonder place; and it shall remove; and nothing shall be impossible unto you.

Matthew 18:19
19 Again I say unto you, that if two of you shall agree on earth as touching anything that they shall ask, it shall be done for them of my Father who is in heaven.

Mark 11:24-25
24 Therefore I say unto you, All things whatsoever ye pray and ask for, believe that ye receive them, and ye shall have them.
25 And whensoever ye stand praying, forgive, if ye have aught against any one; that your Father also who is in heaven may forgive you your trespasses.

Mark 16:17-18
17 And these signs shall accompany them that believe: in my name shall they cast out demons; they shall speak with new tongues;
18 they shall take up serpents, and if they drink any deadly thing, it shall in no wise hurt them; they shall lay hands on the sick, and they shall recover.

Luke 24:25
25 And he said unto them, O foolish men, and slow of heart to believe in all that the prophets have spoken!

John 5:38

38 And ye have not his word abiding in you: for whom he sent, him ye believe not.

John 8:31-34

31 Jesus therefore said to those Jews that had believed him, If ye abide in my word, then are ye truly my disciples;
32 and ye shall know the truth, and the truth shall make you free.
33 They answered unto him, We are Abraham's seed, and have never yet been in bondage to any man: how sayest thou, Ye shall be made free?
34 Jesus answered them, Verily, verily, I say unto you, Every one that committeth sin is the bondservant of sin.

John 14:10-11

10 Believest thou not that I am in the Father, and the Father in me? the words that I say unto you I speak not from myself: but the Father abiding in me doeth his works.
11 Believe me that I am in the Father, and the Father in me: or else believe me for the very works' sake.

John 16:31-33

31 Jesus answered them, Do ye now believe?
32 Behold, the hour cometh, yea, is come, that ye shall be scattered, every man to his own, and shall leave me alone: and yet I am not alone, because the Father is with me.
33 These things have I spoken unto you, that in me ye may have peace. In the world ye have tribulation: but be of good cheer; I have overcome the world.

Acts 15:25-26

25 it seemed good unto us, having come to one accord, to choose out men and send them unto you with our beloved Barnabas and Paul,
26 men that have hazarded their lives for the name of our Lord Jesus Christ.

Acts 20:21
21 testifying both to Jews and to Greeks repentance toward God, and faith toward our Lord Jesus Christ.

Acts 21:13
13 Then Paul answered, What do ye, weeping and breaking my heart? for I am ready not to be bound only, but also to die at Jerusalem for the name of the Lord Jesus.

Romans 10:17
17 So belief cometh of hearing, and hearing by the word of Christ.

Romans 12:3
3 For I say, through the grace that was given me, to every man that is among you, not to think of himself more highly than he ought to think; but to think as to think soberly, according as God hath dealt to each man a measure of faith.

1 Corinthians 2:5
5 that your faith should not stand in the wisdom of men, but in the power of God.

Galatians 3:5
5 He therefore that supplieth to you the Spirit, and worketh miracles among you, doeth he it by the works of the law, or by the hearing of faith?

Hebrews 4:2
2 For indeed we have had good tidings preached unto us, even as also they: but the word of hearing did not profit them, because it was not united by faith with them that heard.

Hebrews 11:1
1 Now faith is assurance of things hoped for, a conviction of things not seen.

Hebrews 12:1-2

1 Therefore let us also, seeing we are compassed about with so great a cloud of witnesses, lay aside every weight, and the sin which doth so easily beset us, and let us run with patience the race that is set before us,

2 looking unto Jesus the author and perfecter of our faith, who for the joy that was set before him endured the cross, despising shame, and hath sat down at the right hand of the throne of God.

James 2:17

17 Even so faith, if it have not works, is dead in itself.

1 Peter 1:3-8

3 Blessed be the God and Father of our Lord Jesus Christ, who according to his great mercy begat us again unto a living hope by the resurrection of Jesus Christ from the dead,

4 unto an inheritance incorruptible, and undefiled, and that fadeth not away, reserved in heaven for you,

5 who by the power of God are guarded through faith unto a salvation ready to be revealed in the last time.

6 Wherein ye greatly rejoice, though now for a little while, if need be, ye have been put to grief in manifold trials,

7 that the proof of your faith, being more precious than gold that perisheth though it is proved by fire, may be found unto praise and glory and honor at the revelation of Jesus Christ:

8 whom not having seen ye love; on whom, though now ye see him not, yet believing, ye rejoice greatly with joy unspeakable and full of glory:

1 John 4:4

4 Ye are of God, my little children, and have overcome them: because greater is he that is in you than he that is in the world.

1 John 5:14-15

14 And this is the boldness which we have toward him, that, if we ask anything according to his will, he heareth us:

15 and if we know that he heareth us whatsoever we ask, we know that we have the petitions which we have asked of him.

Faith in the Power of Jesus' Name

Do you know there is power in Jesus' name? Some people have doubts or choose not to ask anything of the Lord. But if you don't ask, you don't receive. Maybe you have asked and received nothing. Did you have faith that your request would be answered? Maybe you had faith but lost it when you didn't immediately receive what you asked for.

If that's the case, you may need to strengthen your faith. Are you asking for things in God's will? In other words, are you asking for things consistent with His work? Are you living according to His will? Have you allowed Jesus access to your entire life? These are some of the questions to consider. Maybe you have put up barriers in your way which you need to address.

Remember!
When praying scripture, give Jesus permission to search for lies and unbelief and replace them with God's truth.

Acts 4:12   Key Verse

12 And in none other is there salvation: for neither is there any other name under heaven, that is given among men, wherein we must be saved.

Acts 3:16   Key Verse

16 And by faith in his name hath his name made this man strong, whom ye behold and know: yea, the faith which is through him hath given him this perfect soundness in the presence of you all.

1 John 5:13   Key Verse

13 These things have I written unto you, that ye may know that ye have eternal life, even unto you that believe on the name of the Son of God.

Matthew 14:31-32

31 And immediately Jesus stretched forth his hand, and took hold of him, and saith unto him, O thou of little faith, wherefore didst thou doubt?
32 And when they were gone up into the boat, the wind ceased.

John 11:35-44

35 Jesus wept.
36 The Jews therefore said, Behold how he loved him!
37 But some of them said, Could not this man, who opened the eyes of him that was blind, have caused that this man also should not die?
38 Jesus therefore again groaning in himself cometh to the tomb. Now it was a cave, and a stone lay against it.
39 Jesus saith, Take ye away the stone. Martha, the sister of him that was dead, saith unto him, Lord, by this time the body decayeth; for he hath been dead four days.
40 Jesus saith unto her, Said I not unto thee, that, if thou believedst, thou shouldest see the glory of God?
41 So they took away the stone. And Jesus lifted up his eyes, and said, Father, I thank thee that thou heardest me.

42 And I knew that thou hearest me always: but because of the multitude that standeth around I said it, that they may believe that thou didst send me.
43 And when he had thus spoken, he cried with a loud voice, Lazarus, come forth.
44 He that was dead came forth, bound hand and foot with graveclothes; and his face was bound about with a napkin. Jesus saith unto them, Loose him, and let him go.

John 14:12

12 Verily, verily, I say unto you, he that believeth on me, the works that I do shall he do also; and greater works than these shall he do; because I go unto the Father.

John 16:23-26

23 And in that day ye shall ask me no question. Verily, verily, I say unto you, if ye shall ask anything of the Father, he will give it you in my name.
24 Hitherto have ye asked nothing in my name: ask, and ye shall receive, that your joy may be made full.
25 These things have I spoken unto you in dark sayings: the hour cometh, when I shall no more speak unto you in dark sayings, but shall tell you plainly of the Father.
26 In that day ye shall ask in my name: and I say not unto you, that I will pray the Father for you;

Acts 3:6

6 But Peter said, Silver and gold have I none; but what I have, that give I thee. In the name of Jesus Christ of Nazareth, walk.

Acts 4:7

7 And when they had set them in the midst, they inquired, By what power, or in what name, have ye done this?

Acts 4:10

10 be it known unto you all, and to all the people of Israel, that in the name of Jesus Christ of Nazareth, whom ye crucified, whom God raised from the dead, even in him doth this man stand here before you whole.

Acts 5:41-42
41 They therefore departed from the presence of the council, rejoicing that they were counted worthy to suffer dishonor for the Name.
42 And every day, in the temple and at home, they ceased not to teach and to preach Jesus as the Christ.

Acts 13:11-12
11 And now, behold, the hand of the Lord is upon thee, and thou shalt be blind, not seeing the sun for a season. And immediately there fell on him a mist and a darkness; and he went about seeking some to lead him by the hand.
12 Then the proconsul, when he saw what was done, believed, being astonished at the teaching of the Lord.

Acts 14:13
13 And the priest of Jupiter whose temple was before the city, brought oxen and garlands unto the gates, and would have done sacrifice with the multitudes.

Acts 16:18
18 And this she did for many days. But Paul, being sore troubled, turned and said to the spirit, I charge thee in the name of Jesus Christ to come out of her. And it came out that very hour.

Hebrews 4:12-13
12 For the word of God is living, and active, and sharper than any two-edged sword, and piercing even to the dividing of soul and spirit, of both joints and marrow, and quick to discern the thoughts and intents of the heart.
13 And there is no creature that is not manifest in his sight: but all things are naked and laid open before the eyes of him with whom we have to do.

Fear and Anxiety

Fear is the single most problematic, deadly mindset that will plague us if we allow it to pervade our life. Anxiety attacks are usually triggered by unrecognized fear, which is harbored in our memory. Phobias are known fears that exist for no apparent reason.

> *Fear is the single most problematic, deadly mindset that will plague us if we allow it to pervade our life.*

Fear of man is a wide-encompassing problem we will all face, but for many, it can be very destructive. Fear of man is usually fear of what others think of us. Jeremiah 1:8 tells us not to fear the faces of man. Proverbs 1:7 says the fear of the Lord is the beginning of wisdom. In 2 Corinthians 10:5, we are told to take our thoughts captive to the Word of God. So, what should you take more seriously, someone's opinion of you, or God and His Word? What can happen if you place the Lord at number two, or just out of the daily activities of your life?

For many people, a co-dependency on the sinful or evil behaviors of others develops. Some become battered spouses. Or they get drawn into sinful behavior that leads to a whole series of bad decisions and difficult outcomes. This is also true of our children. Peer pressure can influence their poor choices. Where do you think that temptation is incubated? Sometimes it's from the fear of man!

Fear of death is another fear tied into our beliefs of the future. Thoughts of the future can be filled with anxiety if we lack faith or have little hope. Or how about those of us who fear the loss of all our possessions and poverty as a result? If we don't trust that God will provide, we will be fearful. You can see that various topics share common roots. For example, if we fear, we don't trust God. Or if we have anger, we may have to deal with the difficulty of unforgiveness. So as you work on removing fear from your mind or the mind of another person, you need to refill both mind and spirit with trust, love, and other Godly virtues. The truth of God's Word contains virtues that we can use to replace the negative mindsets that plague our lives.

Remember!
When praying scripture, give Jesus permission to search for lies and unbelief and replace them with God's truth.

Psalms 23:4   Key Verse
4 Yea, thou I walk through the valley of the shadow of death, I will fear no evil; for thou art with me; Thy rod and thy staff, they comfort me.

Philippians 4:6-7   Key Verse
6 In nothing be anxious; but in everything by prayer and supplication with thanksgiving let your requests be made known unto God.
7 And the peace of God, which passeth all understanding, shall guard your hearts and your thoughts in Christ Jesus.

Psalms 27:1-3 (War)   Key Verse
1 Jehovah is my light and my salvation; Whom shall I fear? Jehovah is the strength of my life; Of whom shall I be afraid?
2 When evil-doers came upon me to eat up my flesh, Even mine adversaries and my foes, they stumbled and fell.
3 Though a host should encamp against me, My heart shall not fear: Though war should rise against me, Even then will I be confident.

Proverbs 3:24-26   Key Verse
24 When thou liest down, thou shalt not be afraid: Yea, thou shalt lie down, and thy sleep shall be sweet.
25 Be not afraid of sudden fear, Neither of the desolation of the wicked, when it cometh:
26 For Jehovah will be thy confidence, And will keep thy foot from being taken.

Philippians 1:14 (Man)   Key Verse
14 and that most of the brethren in the Lord, being confident through my bonds, are more abundantly bold to speak the word of God without fear.

Genesis 15:1
1 After these things the word of Jehovah came unto Abram in a vision, saying, Fear not, Abram: I am thy shield, and thy exceeding great reward.

Exodus 14:13-14 (Man)
13 And Moses said unto the people, Fear ye not, stand still, and see the salvation of Jehovah, which he will work for you to-day: for the Egyptians whom ye have seen to-day, ye shall see them again no more for ever.
14 Jehovah will fight for you, and ye shall hold your peace.

Deuteronomy 20:4
4 for Jehovah your God is he that goeth with you, to fight for you against your enemies, to save you.

Fear and Anxiety

2 Chronicles 20:15
15 and he said, Hearken ye, all Judah, and ye inhabitants of Jerusalem, and thou king Jehoshaphat: Thus saith Jehovah unto you, Fear not ye, neither be dismayed by reason of this great multitude; for the battle is not yours, but God's.

Job 3:25
25 For the thing which I fear cometh upon me, And that which I am afraid of cometh unto me.

Job 5:20 (Death)
20 In famine he will redeem thee from death; And in war from the power of the sword.

Psalms 4:8 (Sleep)
8 In peace will I both lay me down and sleep; For thou, Jehovah, alone makest me dwell in safety.

Psalms 9:10 (Abandonment)
10 And they that know thy name will put their trust in thee; For thou, Jehovah, hast not forsaken them that seek thee.

Psalms 27:1-2
1 Jehovah is my light and my salvation; Whom shall I fear? Jehovah is the strength of my life; Of whom shall I be afraid?
2 When evil-doers came upon me to eat up my flesh, Even mine adversaries and my foes, they stumbled and fell.

Psalms 27:5-6
5 For in the day of trouble he will keep me secretly in his pavilion: In the covert of his tabernacle will he hide me; He will lift me up upon a rock.
6 And now shall my head be lifted up above mine enemies round about me. And I will offer in his tabernacle sacrifices of joy; I will sing, yea, I will sing praises unto Jehovah.

Psalms 34:4

4 I sought Jehovah, and he answered me, And delivered me from all my fears.

Psalms 37:40

40 And Jehovah helpeth them, and rescueth them; He rescueth them from the wicked, and saveth them, Because they have taken refuge in him.

Psalms 46:1-3

1 God is our refuge and strength, A very present help in trouble.
2 Therefore will we not fear, though the earth do change, And though the mountains be shaken into the heart of the seas;
3 Though the waters thereof roar and be troubled, Though the mountains tremble with the swelling thereof. Selah

Psalms 53:5 (Man)

5 There were they in great fear, where no fear was; For God hath scattered the bones of him that encampeth against thee: Thou hast put them to shame, because of God hath rejected them.

Psalms 56:3-4

3 What time I am afraid, I will put my trust in thee.
4 In God (I will praise his word), In God have I put my trust, I will not be afraid; What can flesh do unto me?

Psalms 60:12

12 Through God we shall do valiantly; For he it is that will tread down our adversaries.

Psalms 112:7-8

7 He shall not be afraid of evil tidings: His heart is fixed, trusting in Jehovah.
8 His heart is established, he shall not be afraid, Until he see his desire upon his adversaries.

Psalms 127:2

2 It is vain for you to rise up early, To take rest late, To eat the bread of toil; For so he giveth unto his beloved sleep.

Psalms 139:9-10

9 If I take the wings of the morning, And dwell in the uttermost parts of the sea;
10 Even there shall thy hand lead me, And thy right hand shall hold me.

Proverbs 1:33 (Demonic)

33 But whoso hearkeneth unto me shall dwell securely, And shall be quiet without fear of evil.

Proverbs 4:13

13 Take fast hold of instruction; Let her not go: Keep her; For she is thy life.

Proverbs 28:1

1 The wicked flee when no man pursueth; But the righteous are bold as a lion.

Proverbs 29:25 (Man)

25 The fear of man bringeth a snare; But whoso putteth his trust in Jehovah shall be safe.

Proverbs 14:32 (Death)

32 The wicked is thrust down in his evil-doing; But the righteous hath a refuge in his death.
Isaiah 8:12
12 Say ye not, A conspiracy, concerning all whereof this people shall say, A conspiracy; neither fear ye their fear, nor be in dread thereof.

Isaiah 29:10

10 For Jehovah hath poured out upon you the spirit of deep sleep, and hath closed your eyes, the prophets; and your heads, the seers, hath he covered.

Isaiah 35:4

4 Say to them that are of a fearful heart, Be strong, fear not: behold, your God will come with vengeance, with the recompense of God; he will come and save you.

Isaiah 41:10-13

10 Fear thou not, for I am with thee; be not dismayed, for I am thy God; I will strengthen thee; yea, I will help thee; yea, I will uphold thee with the right hand of my righteousness.
11 Behold, all they that are incensed against thee shall be put to shame and confounded: they that strive with thee shall be as nothing, and shall perish.
12 Thou shalt seek them, and shalt not find them, even them that contend with thee: they that war against thee shall be as nothing, and as a thing of nought.
13 For I, Jehovah thy God, will hold thy right hand, saying unto thee, Fear not; I will help thee.

Isaiah 54:15

15 Behold, they may gather together, but not by me: whosoever shall gather together against thee shall fall because of thee.

Isaiah 54:17

17 No weapon that is formed against thee shall prosper; and every tongue that shall rise against thee in judgment thou shalt condemn. This is the heritage of the servants of Jehovah, and their righteousness which is of me, saith Jehovah.

Isaiah 51:7-16

7 Hearken unto me, ye that know righteousness, the people in whose heart is my law; fear ye not the reproach of men, neither be ye dismayed at their revilings.
8 For the moth shall eat them up like a garment, and the worm shall eat them like wool; but my righteousness shall be for ever, and my

salvation unto all generations.

9 Awake, awake, put on strength, O arm of Jehovah; awake, as in the days of old, the generations of ancient times. Is it not thou that didst cut Rahab in pieces, that didst pierce the monster?

10 Is it not thou that driedst up the sea, the waters of the great deep; that madest the depths of the sea a way for the redeemed to pass over?

11 And the ransomed of Jehovah shall return, and come with singing unto Zion; and everlasting joy shall be upon their heads: they shall obtain gladness and joy; and sorrow and sighing shall flee away.

12 I, even I, am he that comforteth you: who art thou, that thou art afraid of man that shall die, and of the son of man that shall be made as grass;

13 and hast forgotten Jehovah thy Maker, that stretched forth the heavens, and laid the foundations of the earth; and fearest continually all the day because of the fury of the oppressor, when he maketh ready to destroy? and where is the fury of the oppressor?

14 The captive exile shall speedily be loosed; and he shall not die and go down into the pit, neither shall his bread fail.

15 For I am Jehovah thy God, who stirreth up the sea, so that the waves thereof roar: Jehovah of hosts is his name.

16 And I have put my words in thy mouth, and have covered thee in the shadow of my hand, that I may plant the heavens, and lay the foundations of the earth, and say unto Zion, Thou art my people.

Isaiah 59:19

19 So shall they fear the name of Jehovah from the west, and his glory from the rising of the sun; for he will come as a rushing stream, which the breath of Jehovah driveth.

Jeremiah 1:8 (Man)

8 Be not afraid because of them; for I am with thee to deliver thee, saith Jehovah.

Jeremiah 39:17-18

17 But I will deliver thee in that day, saith Jehovah; and thou shalt

not be given into the hand of the men of whom thou art afraid.
18 For I will surely save thee, and thou shalt not fall by the sword, but thy life shall be for a prey unto thee; because thou hast put thy trust in me, saith Jehovah.

Hosea 13:14 (Death)
14 I will ransom them from the power of Sheol; I will redeem them from death: O death, where are thy plagues? O Sheol, where is thy destruction? repentance shall be hid from mine eyes.

Haggai 2:5
5 according to the word that I covenanted with you when ye came out of Egypt, and my Spirit abode among you: fear ye not.
Hebrews 1:12 (ASV) (Old Age)
12 And as a mantle shalt thou roll them up, As a garment, and they shall be changed: But thou art the same, And thy years shall not fail.

Matthew 6:31-34 (Provision)
31 Be not therefore anxious, saying, What shall we eat? or, What shall we drink? or, Wherewithal shall we be clothed?
32 For after all these things do the Gentiles seek; for your heavenly Father knoweth that ye have need of all these things.
33 But seek ye first his kingdom, and his righteousness; and all these things shall be added unto you.
34 Be not therefore anxious for the morrow: for the morrow will be anxious for itself. Sufficient unto the day is the evil thereof.

Matthew 10:26-28 (Fear of Man)
26 Fear them not therefore: for there is nothing covered, that shall not be revealed; and hid, that shall not be known.
27 What I tell you in the darkness, speak ye in the light; and what ye hear in the ear, proclaim upon the house-tops.
28 And be not afraid of them that kill the body, but are not able to kill the soul: but rather fear him who is able to destroy both soul and body in hell.

Matthew 14:27-31

27 But straightway Jesus spake unto them, saying Be of good cheer; it is I; be not afraid.
28 And Peter answered him and said, Lord, if it be thou, bid me come unto the upon the waters.
29 And he said, Come. And Peter went down from the boat, and walked upon the waters to come to Jesus.
30 But when he saw the wind, he was afraid; and beginning to sink, he cried out, saying, Lord, save me.
31 And immediately Jesus stretched forth his hand, and took hold of him, and saith unto him, O thou of little faith, wherefore didst thou doubt?

Matthew 16:2

2 But he answered and said unto them, When it is evening, ye say, It will be fair weather: for the heaven is red.

Matthew 16:17-18 (Death)

17 And Jesus answered and said unto him, Blessed art thou, Simon Bar-jonah: for flesh and blood hath not revealed it unto thee, but my Father who is in heaven.
18 And I also say unto thee, that thou art Peter, and upon this rock I will build my church; and the gates of Hades shall not prevail against it.

Matthew 16:23 (Man)

23 But he turned, and said unto Peter, Get thee behind me, Satan: thou art a stumbling-block unto me: for thou mindest not the things of God, but the things of men.

Mark 4:39-41

39 And he awoke, and rebuked the wind, and said unto the sea, Peace, be still. And the wind ceased, and there was a great calm.
40 And he said unto them, Why are ye fearful? have ye not yet faith?
41 And they feared exceedingly, and said one to another, Who then

is this, that even the wind and the sea obey him?

Luke 1:74
74 To grant unto us that we being delivered out of the hand of our enemies Should serve him without fear,

Luke 10:19
19 Behold, I have given you authority to tread upon serpents and scorpions, and over all the power of the enemy: and nothing shall in any wise hurt you.

Luke 12:22-26
22 And he said unto his disciples, Therefore I say unto you, Be not anxious for your life, what ye shall eat; nor yet for your body, what ye shall put on.
23 For the life is more than the food, and the body than the raiment.
24 Consider the ravens, that they sow not, neither reap; which have no store-chamber nor barn; and God feedeth them: of how much more value are ye than the birds!
25 And which of you by being anxious can add a cubit unto the measure of his life?
26 If then ye are not able to do even that which is least, why are ye anxious concerning the rest?

Luke 12:32
32 Fear not, little flock; for it is your Father's good pleasure to give you the kingdom.

Luke 13:16
16 And ought not this woman, being a daughter of Abraham, whom Satan had bound, lo, these eighteen years, to have been loosed from this bond on the day of the sabbath?

John 3:15 (Death)
15 that whosoever believeth may in him have eternal life.

John 6:20 (Death)
20 But he saith unto them, It is I; be not afraid.

John 16:32
32 Behold, the hour cometh, yea, is come, that ye shall be scattered, every man to his own, and shall leave me alone: and yet I am not alone, because the Father is with me.

Acts 9:31
31 So the church throughout all Judaea and Galilee and Samaria had peace, being edified; and, walking in the fear of the Lord and in the comfort of the Holy Spirit, was multiplied.

Romans 8:15
15 For ye received not the spirit of bondage again unto fear; but ye received the spirit of adoption, whereby we cry, Abba, Father.

Romans 8:37
37 Nay, in all these things we are more than conquerors through him that loved us.

Romans 8:38-39 (Death)
38 For I am persuaded, that neither death, nor life, nor angels, nor principalities, nor things present, nor things to come, nor powers,
39 nor height, nor depth, nor any other creature, shall be able to separate us from the love of God, which is in Christ Jesus our Lord.

1 Corinthians 15:57
57 but thanks be to God, who giveth us the victory through our Lord Jesus Christ.

2 Corinthians 2:14
14 But thanks be unto God, who always leadeth us in triumph in Christ, and maketh manifest through us the savor of his knowledge in every place.

Galatians 1:10 (Man)
10 For am I now seeking the favor of men, or of God? or am I striving to please men? if I were still pleasing men, I should not be a servant of Christ.

Philippians 1:21 (Death)
21 For to me to live is Christ, and to die is gain.

2 Timothy 1:6-7 (Boldness)
6 For which cause I put thee in remembrance that thou stir up the gift of God, which is in thee through the laying on of my hands.
7 For God gave us not a spirit of fearfulness; but of power and love and discipline.

Hebrews 2:14-15 (Death)
14 Since then the children are sharers in flesh and blood, he also himself in like manner partook of the same; that through death he might bring to nought him that had the power of death, that is, the devil;
15 and might deliver all them who through fear of death were all their lifetime subject to bondage.

Hebrews 2:15 (Death)
15 and might deliver all them who through fear of death were all their lifetime subject to bondage.

Hebrews 13:6
6 So that with good courage we say, The Lord is my helper; I will not fear: What shall man do unto me?

1 Peter 3:14
14 But even if ye should suffer for righteousness' sake, blessed are ye: and fear not their fear, neither be troubled;

1 Peter 5:6-7
6 Humble yourselves therefore under the mighty hand of God, that

he may exalt you in due time;
7 casting all your anxiety upon him, because he careth for you.

1 John 4:4
4 Ye are of God, my little children, and have overcome them: because greater is he that is in you than he that is in the world.

1 John 4:18
18 There is no fear in love: but perfect love casteth out fear, because fear hath punishment; and he that feareth is not made perfect in love.

Revelation 2:10
10 Fear not the things which thou art about to suffer: behold, the devil is about to cast some of you into prison, that ye may be tried; and ye shall have tribulation ten days. Be thou faithful unto death, and I will give thee the crown of life.

Forgiveness

The idea of forgiveness is more than just mental ascension, rather, it is an action—the act of forgiving. It is also more than just knowing we should forgive. Actually doing it—forgiving—may be one of the most difficult things you will ever do because it goes against what you might feel. However, choosing not to forgive is like having the talons of a giant bird hooking into you. By repressing our thoughts of forgiveness, we may seem to do okay, at least for a time, and then those emotions surface again.

Many times we assume the blame of what was done to us. Of course, this will affect how we perceive ourselves. We could end up living according to self-imposed identities of shame, guilt, self-hate, unworthiness, and so forth when we don't need to. It is a paradox that our offender still controls us years after the offense, yet only we can release this hook.

God's truth about forgiveness will help us to forgive. The offender may have hurt us numerous times, so we may find that we will have to continue to forgive our offender as different events are brought to our mind. This is a critical point; do not assume one prayer of forgiveness has totally released you. You may need to forgive a person many times for offenses as you recall various memories. Anger can be attached to these painful memories, which is why you must forgive that person for each offense in order for peace to come into your life. Peter asked Jesus if forgiving someone seven times would be enough. Jesus replied *"70 times seven."*

> *You may need to forgive a person many times for each offense against you.*

Another scenario I hear is "this person is still hurting me, so how can I forgive." It may be in words, controlling behavior, or in other deeds that this plays out. First, you will always be in bondage to that person until you release them. You can't control what others do, only yourself. It is up to you and your cooperation with Jesus to set you free. If you seek and receive emotional healing for all offenses and wounds of the past, then that person can't continue to hurt you. Their hurtful behavior will just slide off you while you remain in perfect peace. Sound incredible? It certainly does, but it's true.

You will then be able to look at this person with compassion, just like Jesus, and recognize that they are acting the way they are toward you because of their wounds and strongholds. Your Godly light will shine, and they will see from the change in your life that there is hope for theirs.

Another thing I hear is, "no way can I forgive them, the event was too horrific." But just as God forgives all sin, so must we. Our bodies cannot withstand the burden of bearing anger, bitterness, and resentment. These feelings can only be released through forgiveness. Living long

> *Our bodies cannot withstand the burden of bearing anger, bitterness, and resentment.*

term with unforgiveness wears the body down, leads to physical and mental afflictions, and results in all kinds of negative ramifications in your life. Although Jesus suffered on the cross for you, by choosing not to forgive you choose to suffer again for the things Jesus has already suffered for on your behalf. In effect, you are negating the workings of His sacrifice in your life.

Remember!
When praying scripture, give Jesus permission to search for lies and unbelief and replace them with God's truth.

1 John 1:9   Key Verse
9 If we confess our sins, he is faithful and righteous to forgive us our sins, and to cleanse us from all unrighteousness.

Luke 6:35-38   Key Verse
35 But love your enemies, and do them good, and lend, never despairing; and your reward shall be great, and ye shall be sons of the Most High: for he is kind toward the unthankful and evil.
36 Be ye merciful, even as your Father is merciful.
37 And judge not, and ye shall not be judged: and condemn not, and ye shall not be condemned: release, and ye shall be released:
38 give, and it shall be given unto you; good measure, pressed down, shaken together, running over, shall they give into your bosom. For with what measure ye mete it shall be measured to you again.

Matthew 6:14   Key Verse
14 For if ye forgive men their trespasses, your heavenly Father will also forgive you.

Psalms 66:18   Key Verse

18 If I regard iniquity in my heart, The Lord will not hear:

Leviticus 26:40-42

40 And they shall confess their iniquity, and the iniquity of their fathers, in their trespass which they trespassed against me, and also that, because they walked contrary unto me,
41 I also walked contrary unto them, and brought them into the land of their enemies: if then their uncircumcised heart be humbled, and they then accept of the punishment of their iniquity;
42 then will I remember my covenant with Jacob; and also my covenant with Isaac, and also my covenant with Abraham will I remember; and I will remember the land.

Psalms 22:1-5

1 My God, my God, why hast thou forsaken me? Why art thou so far from helping me, and from the words of my groaning?
2 O my God, I cry in the daytime, but thou answerest not; And in the night season, and am not silent.
3 But thou art holy, O thou that inhabitest the praises of Israel.
4 Our fathers trusted in thee: They trusted, and thou didst deliver them.
5 They cried unto thee, and were delivered: They trusted in thee, and were not put to shame.

Psalms 51:14

14 Deliver me from bloodguiltiness, O God, thou God of my salvation; And my tongue shall sing aloud of thy righteousness.

Proverbs 6:2-3

2 Thou art snared with the words of thy mouth, Thou art taken with the words of thy mouth.
3 Do this now, my son, and deliver thyself, Seeing thou art come into the hand of thy neighbor: Go, humble thyself, and importune thy neighbor;

Proverbs 20:22
22 Say not thou, I will recompense evil: Wait for Jehovah, and he will save thee.

Isaiah 1:15
15 And when ye spread forth your hands, I will hide mine eyes from you; yea, when ye make many prayers, I will not hear: your hands are full of blood.

Isaiah 43:25
25 I, even I, am he that blotteth out thy transgressions for mine own sake; and I will not remember thy sins.

Isaiah 59:2
2 but your iniquities have separated between you and your God, and your sins have hid his face from you, so that he will not hear.

Ezekiel 33:13
13 When I say to the righteous, that he shall surely live; if he trust to his righteousness, and commit iniquity, none of his righteous deeds shall be remembered; but in his iniquity that he hath committed, therein shall he die.

Matthew 5:44-45
44 but I say unto you, love your enemies, and pray for them that persecute you;
45 that ye may be sons of your Father who is in heaven: for he maketh his sun to rise on the evil and the good, and sendeth rain on the just and the unjust.

Matthew 6:15
15 But if ye forgive not men their trespasses, neither will your Father forgive your trespasses.

Matthew 12:37
37 For by thy words thou shalt be justified, and by thy words thou

shalt be condemned.

Matthew 18:21-22
21 Then came Peter and said to him, Lord, how oft shall my brother sin against me, and I forgive him? until seven times?
22 Jesus saith unto him, I say not unto thee, Until seven times; but, Until seventy times seven.

Mark 11:25
25 And whensoever ye stand praying, forgive, if ye have aught against any one; that your Father also who is in heaven may forgive you your trespasses.

Luke 15:20
20 And he arose, and came to his father. But while he was yet afar off, his father saw him, and was moved with compassion, and ran, and fell on his neck, and kissed him.

Luke 23:34
34 And Jesus said, Father, forgive them; for they know not what they do. And parting his garments among them, they cast lots.

2 Corinthians 2:10-11
10 But to whom ye forgive anything, I forgive also: for what I also have forgiven, if I have forgiven anything, for your sakes have I forgiven it in the presence of Christ;
11 that no advantage may be gained over us by Satan: for we are not ignorant of his devices.

Colossians 2:12-15
12 having been buried with him in baptism, wherein ye were also raised with him through faith in the working of God, who raised him from the dead.
13 And you, being dead through your trespasses and the uncircumcision of your flesh, you, I say, did he make alive together with him, having forgiven us all our trespasses;

14 having blotted out the bond written in ordinances that was against us, which was contrary to us: and he hath taken it out that way, nailing it to the cross;

15 having despoiled the principalities and the powers, he made a show of them openly, triumphing over them in it.

Colossians 3:5

5 Put to death therefore your members which are upon the earth: fornication, uncleanness, passion, evil desire, and covetousness, which is idolatry;

Hebrews 9:22

22 And according to the law, I may almost say, all things are cleansed with blood, and apart from shedding of blood there is no remission.

Hebrews 12:15

15 looking carefully lest there be any man that falleth short of the grace of God; lest any root of bitterness springing up trouble you, and thereby the many be defiled;

James 5:20

20 let him know, that he who converteth a sinner from the error of his way shall save a soul from death, and shall cover a multitude of sins.

God's Grace

One neat thing about being a Christian is there is no list of things we must do to get to heaven; our works won't get us there. That separates Christians from followers of other religions. All you have to do is accept Jesus in faith, and allow Jesus to cleanse you of your sins as you seek His forgiveness and turn away from sin.

Are you having trouble receiving God's grace? Maybe you need to come to God for the first time in your life, or perhaps you are finding the need to reaffirm your faith. Let God's Word sink into all aspects of your life with the truth of this grace. It is one thing to know God's grace on an intellectual level, but it's another thing to experience it. Knowing His grace on an experiential level—through a personal relationship with God—gives us the confidence to live daily with hope for the future. Life shouldn't be a continuous rollercoaster ride.

> *It is one thing to know God's grace on an intellectual level, but it's another thing to experience it.*

Remember!
When praying scripture, give Jesus permission to search for lies and unbelief and replace them with God's truth.

Romans 5:2   Key Verse
2 through whom also we have had our access by faith into this grace wherein we stand; and we rejoice in hope of the glory of God.

Romans 6:14   Key Verse
14 For sin shall not have dominion over you: for ye are not under law, but under grace.

Titus 2:11   Key Verse
11 For the grace of God hath appeared, bringing salvation to all men,

Matthew 9:37-38
37 Then saith he unto his disciples, The harvest indeed is plenteous, but the laborers are few.
38 Pray ye therefore the Lord of the harvest, that he send forth laborers into his harvest.

Luke 11:36
36 If therefore thy whole body be full of light, having no part dark, it shall be wholly full of light, as when the lamp with its bright shining doth give thee light.

Luke 13:5
5 I tell you, Nay: but, except ye repent, ye shall all likewise perish.

John 1:12
12 But as many as received him, to them gave he the right to become children of God, even to them that believe on his name:
Revelation 3:19 (ASV)

19 As many as I love, I reprove and chasten: be zealous therefore, and repent.

John 1:17
17 For the law was given through Moses; grace and truth came through Jesus Christ.

John 4:14
14 but whosoever drinketh of the water that I shall give him shall never thirst; but the water that I shall give him shall become in him a well of water springing up unto eternal life.

Acts 4:12
12 And in none other is there salvation: for neither is there any other name under heaven, that is given among men, wherein we must be saved.

Acts 15:11
11 But we believe that we shall be saved through the grace of the Lord Jesus, in like manner as they.

Acts 16:31
31 And they said, Believe on the Lord Jesus, and thou shalt be saved, thou and thy house.

Acts 22:16
16 And now why tarriest thou? arise, and be baptized, and wash away thy sins, calling on his name.

Romans 3:21-26
21 But now apart from the law a righteousness of God hath been manifested, being witnessed by the law and the prophets, being witnessed by the law and the prophets;
22 even the righteousness of God through faith in Jesus Christ unto all them that believe; for there is no distinction;
23 for all have sinned, and fall short of the glory of God;

24 being justified freely by his grace through the redemption that is in Christ Jesus:
25 whom God set forth to be a propitiation, through faith, in his blood, to show his righteousness because of the passing over of the sins done aforetime, in the forbearance of God;
26 for the showing, I say, of his righteousness at this present season: that he might himself be just, and the justifier of him that hath faith in Jesus.

Romans 5:15

15 But not as the trespass, so also is the free gift. For if by the trespass of the one the many died, much more did the grace of God, and the gift by the grace of the one man, Jesus Christ, abound unto the many.

Romans 5:17

17 For if, by the trespass of the one, death reigned through the one; much more shall they that receive the abundance of grace and of the gift of righteousness reign in life through the one, even Jesus Christ.

Romans 5:20-21

20 And the law came in besides, that the trespass might abound; but where sin abounded, grace did abound more exceedingly:
21 that, as sin reigned in death, even so might grace reign through righteousness unto eternal life through Jesus Christ our Lord.

Romans 6:23

23 For the wages of sin is death; but the free gift of God is eternal life in Christ Jesus our Lord.

Romans 7:1

1 Or are ye ignorant, brethren (for I speak to men who know the law), that the law hath dominion over a man for so long time as he liveth?

Romans 10:9-10

9 because if thou shalt confess with thy mouth Jesus as Lord, and shalt believe in thy heart that God raised him from the dead, thou shalt be saved:
10 for with the heart man believeth unto righteousness; and with the mouth confession is made unto salvation.

Romans 10:13

13 for, Whosoever shall call upon the name of the Lord shall be saved.

Romans 11:6

6 But if it is by grace, it is no more of works: otherwise grace is no more grace.

1 Corinthians 15:21

21 For since by man came death, by man came also the resurrection of the dead.

2 Corinthians 5:17

17 Wherefore if any man is in Christ, he is a new creature: the old things are passed away; behold, they are become new.

2 Corinthians 8:9

9 For ye know the grace of our Lord Jesus Christ, that, though he was rich, yet for your sakes he became poor, that ye through his poverty might become rich.

2 Corinthians 9:8

8 And God is able to make all grace abound unto you; that ye, having always all sufficiency in everything, may abound unto every good work:

Galatians 3:13

13 Christ redeemed us from the curse of the law, having become a curse for us; for it is written, Cursed is every one that hangeth on a tree:

Ephesians 1:7
7 in whom we have our redemption through his blood, the forgiveness of our trespasses, according to the riches of his grace,

Ephesians 2:8-9
8 for by grace have ye been saved through faith; and that not of yourselves, it is the gift of God;
9 not of works, that no man should glory.

Colossians 3:16
16 Let the word of Christ dwell in you richly; in all wisdom teaching and admonishing one another with psalms and hymns and spiritual songs, singing with grace in your hearts unto God.

Colossians 4:6
6 Let your speech be always with grace, seasoned with salt, that ye may know how ye ought to answer each one.

Titus 3:7
7 that, being justified by his grace, we might be made heirs according to the hope of eternal life.

Hebrews 4:16
16 Let us therefore draw near with boldness unto the throne of grace, that we may receive mercy, and may find grace to help us in time of need.

1 John 1:9
9 If we confess our sins, he is faithful and righteous to forgive us our sins, and to cleanse us from all unrighteousness.

1 John 2:1
1 My little children, these things write I unto you that ye may not sin. And if any man sin, we have an Advocate with the Father, Jesus Christ the righteous:

Guilt and Shame

Guilt and shame can be positive feelings when they prevent us from taking negative actions. Our conscience was designed by God and He doesn't want us to live a shameful life; He wants us to be free. When we seek and receive forgiveness for our sins, our lives become clean. God's forgiveness includes the removal of guilt and shame. If you feel shame, then quite likely you need to deal with sin issues.

There is another source of shame, however. It occurs when an offense (sin) is committed against us. This can happen when a child is sexually abused, but it's not limited to this situation. The abused person is made to feel shameful, dirty, and usually worse. This is a lie that Satan will use to torment a person. Jesus wants to remove these lies and set you free. Also in this situation, a person may

> *Once we have asked for God's forgiveness for something we've done in the past, we won't continue feeling shameful and guilty.*

feel guilty, as if they somehow caused the event.

Once we have asked for God's forgiveness for something we've done in the past, we won't continue feeling shameful and guilty. If we still feel this way, we need Jesus to show us why. Know that He will accept our shame and guilt. Satan uses shame and guilt to keep us from living a victorious life.

> **Remember!**
> When praying scripture, give Jesus permission to search for lies and unbelief and replace them with God's truth.

2 Timothy 1:12   Key Verse
12 For which cause I suffer also these things: yet I am not ashamed; for I know him whom I have believed, and I am persuaded that he is able to guard that which I have committed unto him against that day.

Acts 13:38-39   Key Verse
38 Be it known unto you therefore, brethren, that through this man is proclaimed unto you remission of sins:
39 and by him every one that believeth is justified from all things, from which ye could not be justified by the law of Moses.

Isaiah 50:7   Key Verse
7 For the Lord Jehovah will help me; therefore have I not been confounded: therefore have I set my face like a flint, and I know that I shall not be put to shame.

Psalms 19:12-14
12 Who can discern his errors? Clear thou me from hidden faults.

13 Keep back thy servant also from presumptuous sins; Let them not have dominion over me: Then shall I be upright, And I shall be clear from great transgression.
14 Let the words of my mouth and the meditation of my heart Be acceptable in thy sight, O Jehovah, my rock, and my redeemer.

Psalms 103:12
12 As far as the east is from the west, So far hath he removed our transgressions from us.

Psalms 119:6
6 Then shall I not be put to shame, When I have respect unto all thy commandments.

Psalms 119:80
80 Let my heart be perfect in thy statutes, That I be not put to shame.

Isaiah 6:7
7 and he touched my mouth with it, and said, Lo, this hath touched thy lips; and thine iniquity is taken away, and thy sin forgiven.

Isaiah 43:25
25 I, even I, am he that blotteth out thy transgressions for mine own sake; and I will not remember thy sins.

Isaiah 53:6
6 All we like sheep have gone astray; we have turned every one to his own way; and Jehovah hath laid on him the iniquity of us all.

Isaiah 55:7
7 let the wicked forsake his way, and the unrighteous man his thoughts; and let him return unto Jehovah, and he will have mercy upon him; and to our God, for he will abundantly pardon.

Jeremiah 33:8

8 And I will cleanse them from all their iniquity, whereby they have sinned against me; and I will pardon all their iniquities, whereby they have sinned against me, and whereby they have transgressed against me.

Joel 2:6

6 At their presence the peoples are in anguish; all faces are waxed pale.

Romans 5:5

5 and hope putteth not to shame; because the love of God hath been shed abroad in our hearts through the Holy Spirit which was given unto us.

Romans 8:1-2

1 There is therefore now no condemnation to them that are in Christ Jesus.
2 For the law of the Spirit of life in Christ Jesus made me free from the law of sin and of death.

Romans 9:33 (ASV)

33 even as it is written, Behold, I lay in Zion a stone of stumbling and a rock of offence: And he that believeth on him shall not be put to shame.

Romans 10:11 (ASV)

11 For the scripture saith, Whosoever believeth on him shall not be put to shame.

Romans 16:20

20 And the God of peace shall bruise Satan under your feet shortly. The grace of our Lord Jesus Christ be with you.

2 Corinthians 13:13

13 All the saints salute you.

Galatians 3:11

11 Now that no man is justified by the law before God, is evident: for, The righteous shall live by faith;

Galatians 3:19

19 What then is the law? It was added because of transgressions, till the seed should come to whom the promise hath been made; and it was ordained through angels by the hand of a mediator.

Galatians 3:22

22 But the scriptures shut up all things under sin, that the promise by faith in Jesus Christ might be given to them that believe.

Galatians 3:24

24 So that the law is become our tutor to bring us unto Christ, that we might be justified by faith.

Galatians 5:4

4 Ye are severed from Christ, ye would be justified by the law; ye are fallen away from grace.

Colossians 1:22

22 yet now hath he reconciled in the body of his flesh through death, to present you holy and without blemish and unreproveable before him:

2 Timothy 2:15

15 Give diligence to present thyself approved unto God, a workman that needeth not to be ashamed, handling aright the word of truth.

Hebrews 8:12

12 For I will be merciful to their iniquities, And their sins will I remember no more.

1 Peter 4:16

16 but if a man suffer as a Christian, let him not be ashamed; but let him glorify God in this name.

1 John 1:7
7 but if we walk in the light, as he is in the light, we have fellowship one with another, and the blood of Jesus his Son cleanseth us from all sin.

1 John 1:9
9 If we confess our sins, he is faithful and righteous to forgive us our sins, and to cleanse us from all unrighteousness.

1 John 2:12
12 I write unto you, my little children, because your sins are forgiven you for his name's sake.

Healing, Wounds, Disease, and Injury

There are many references to God's healing in the Old and New Testaments. During Jesus' three-year ministry, many were healed. At times, He told people their faith healed them. Jesus said in Matthew 17:20-21, "*Because of your unbelief for assuredly, I say to you, if you have faith of a mustard seed, you will say to this mountain 'Move from here to there', and it will move; nothing will be impossible for you. However, this kind* (of unbelief) *does not go out except by prayer and fasting.*" In this case, prayer and fasting was needed to remove the unbelief and gain the faith to cast out a demon.

Another time, Jesus put mud and spit in a man's eye and then the man could see. It seems that Jesus had no hard and fast method of healing, but the end result is that He did, in fact, heal. In examining the conditions related to all of His healings, one common denominator is apparent: the person

> *The person being healed usually had to do something—respond with an act of faith or obedience.*

being healed usually had to do something—respond with an act of faith or obedience. We can hear the faith of the Centurion who told Jesus to speak the word only and my servant will be healed. And we can see the faith of the sick man with palsy, whose friends lowered him down in a bed to Jesus.

Sometimes Jesus told the healed to sin no more, which implies that sin was the cause and further sin would bring a relapse. If that model applies to us, we may need to be forgiven and repent from our sin in order to gain and maintain our healing. We may have to release our fear, guilt, shame, or anger toward God.

Emotional wounds that are afflicted upon us during our childhood may cause us to see and live life through a distorted lens. We make choices based on this distortion. We use drugs and alcohol to relieve pain, but the painkillers inflict greater harm on us in the long run. We may feel unworthy, unloved, afraid, rejected, or abandoned, all of which are feelings that are destructive to relationships.

> *These unfulfilled needs left by those old wounds just seem to draw us to where we shouldn't go.*

These unfulfilled needs left by those old wounds just seem to draw us to where we shouldn't go. That could mean different places for different people. So, how do we find out what unfulfilled needs are tempting us? We ask the Counselor. We may not get the answers all at once, but as we shed some of our negative strongholds, we are able to get closer to Jesus and begin to hear what He wants us to know.

Healing our physical body may come out of reconciling our strongholds and emotional wounds. Sometimes, Jesus simply heals us and we are left with no understanding of why. We just need to accept what He does for us as a gift.

Remember!
When praying scripture, give Jesus permission to search for lies and unbelief and replace them with God's truth.

James 5:16   Key Verse
16 Confess therefore your sins one to another, and pray one for another, that ye may be healed. The supplication of a righteous man availeth much in its working.

Psalms 41:4   Key Verse
4 I said, O Jehovah, have mercy upon me: Heal my soul; For I have sinned against thee.

Leviticus 17:11
11 For the life of the flesh is in the blood; and I have given it to you upon the altar to make atonement for your souls: for it is the blood that maketh atonement by reason of the life.

Psalms 6:2-3
2 Have mercy upon me, O Jehovah; for I am withered away: O Jehovah, heal me; for my bones are troubled.
3 My soul also is sore troubled: And thou, O Jehovah, how long?

Psalms 30:2
2 O Jehovah my God, I cried unto thee, and thou hast healed me.

Psalms 51:17
17 The sacrifices of God are a broken spirit: A broken and contrite heart, O God, thou wilt not despise.

Psalms 80:19
19 Turn us again, O Jehovah God of hosts; Cause thy face to shine, and we shall be saved.

Psalms 139:23-24
23 Search me, O God, and know my heart: Try me, and know my thoughts;
24 And see if there be any wicked way in me, And lead me in the way everlasting.

Psalms 138:8
8 Jehovah will perfect that which concerneth me: Thy lovingkindness, O Jehovah, endureth for ever; Forsake not the works of thine own hands.

Psalms 147:3 (Broken Heart)
3 He healeth the broken in heart, And bindeth up their wounds.

Isaiah 53:5
5 But he was wounded for our transgressions, he was bruised for our iniquities; the chastisement of our peace was upon him; and with his stripes we are healed.

Jeremiah 30:19
19 And out of them shall proceed thanksgiving and the voice of them that make merry: and I will multiply them, and they shall not be few; I will also glorify them, and they shall not be small.

Jeremiah 33:16
16 In those days shall Judah be saved, and Jerusalem shall dwell safely; and this is the name whereby she shall be called: Jehovah our righteousness.

Ezekiel 36:26
26 A new heart also will I give you, and a new spirit will I put within you; and I will take away the stony heart out of your flesh, and I will give you a heart of flesh.

Joel 2:25
25 And I will restore to you the years that the locust hath eaten, the

canker-worm, and the caterpillar, and the palmer-worm, my great army which I sent among you.

Mark 2:17
17 And when Jesus heard it, he saith unto them, They that are whole have no need of a physician, but they that are sick: I came not to call the righteous, but sinners.

Mark 3:10
10 for he had healed many; insomuch that as many as had plagues pressed upon him that they might touch him.

Mark 10:52
52 And Jesus said unto him, Go thy way; thy faith hath made thee whole. And straightway he received his sight, and followed him in the way.

John 7:37-38
37 Now on the last day, the great day of the feast, Jesus stood and cried, saying, If any man thirst, let him come unto me and drink.
38 He that believeth on me, as the scripture hath said, from within him shall flow rivers of living water.

John 8:36
36 If therefore the Son shall make you free, ye shall be free indeed.

John 15:1-2
1 I am the true vine, and my Father is the husbandman.
2 Every branch in me that beareth not fruit, he taketh it away: and every branch that beareth fruit, he cleanseth it, that it may bear more fruit.

John 17:17
17 Sanctify them in the truth: thy word is truth.

Romans 6:23
23 For the wages of sin is death; but the free gift of God is eternal life in Christ Jesus our Lord.

2 Corinthians 3:17
17 Now the Lord is the Spirit: and where the Spirit of the Lord is, there is liberty.

Ephesians 2:14
14 For he is our peace, who made both one, and brake down the middle wall of partition,

Ephesians 4:31
31 Let all bitterness, and wrath, and anger, and clamor, and railing, be put away from you, with all malice:

Hebrews 12:15
15 looking carefully lest there be any man that falleth short of the grace of God; lest any root of bitterness springing up trouble you, and thereby the many be defiled;

1 Peter 2:24
24 who his own self bare our sins in his body upon the tree, that we, having died unto sins, might live unto righteousness; by whose stripes ye were healed.

1 John 1:7
7 but if we walk in the light, as he is in the light, we have fellowship one with another, and the blood of Jesus his Son cleanseth us from all sin.

1 John 3:21-22
21 Beloved, if our heart condemn us not, we have boldness toward God;
22 and whatsoever we ask we receive of him, because we keep his commandments and do the things that are pleasing in his sight.

1 John 4:4
4 Ye are of God, my little children, and have overcome them: because greater is he that is in you than he that is in the world.

Revelation 21:5-6
5 And he that sitteth on the throne said, Behold, I make all things new. And he saith, Write: for these words are faithful and true.
6 And he said unto me, They are come to pass. I am the Alpha and the Omega, the beginning and the end. I will give unto him that is athirst of the fountain of the water of life freely.

Revelation 22:1-3
1 And he showed me a river of water of life, bright as crystal, proceeding out of the throne of God and of the Lamb,
2 in the midst of the street thereof. And on this side of the river and on that was the tree of life, bearing twelve manner of fruits, yielding its fruit every month: and the leaves of the tree were for the healing of the nations.
3 And there shall be no curse any more: and the throne of God and of the Lamb shall be therein: and his servants shall serve him;

Physical Healing

Psalms 107:20   Key Verse
20 He sendeth his word, and healeth them, And delivereth them from their destructions.

Matthew 4:23   Key Verse
23 And Jesus went about in all Galilee, teaching in their synagogues, and preaching the gospel of the kingdom, and healing all manner of disease and all manner of sickness among the people.

Exodus 15:26
26 and he said, If thou wilt diligently hearken to the voice of Jehovah thy God, and wilt do that which is right in his eyes, and wilt give ear to his commandments, and keep all his statutes, I will put none of

the diseases upon thee, which I have put upon the Egyptians: for I am Jehovah that healeth thee.

Exodus 23:25

25 And ye shall serve Jehovah your God, and he will bless thy bread, and thy water; and I will take sickness away from the midst of thee.

Psalms 103:2-3

2 Bless Jehovah, O my soul, And forget not all his benefits:
3 Who forgiveth all thine iniquities; Who healeth all thy diseases;

Proverbs 4:20-22

20 My son, attend to my words; Incline thine ear unto my sayings.
21 Let them not depart from thine eyes; Keep them in the midst of thy heart.
22 For they are life unto those that find them, And health to all their flesh.

Proverbs 14:27

27 The fear of Jehovah is a fountain of life, That one may depart from the snares of death.

Ezekiel 18:26

26 When the righteous man turneth away from his righteousness, and committeth iniquity, and dieth therein; in his iniquity that he hath done shall he die.

Malachi 4:2

2 But unto you that fear my name shall the sun of righteousness arise with healing in its wings; and ye shall go forth, and gambol as calves of the stall.

Matthew 8:16-17

16 And when even was come, they brought unto him many possessed with demons: and he cast out the spirits with a word, and healed all

that were sick:
17 that it might be fulfilled which was spoken through Isaiah the prophet, saying: Himself took our infirmities, and bare our diseases.

Matthew 9:22
22 But Jesus turning and seeing her said, Daughter, be of good cheer; thy faith hath made thee whole. And the woman was made whole from that hour.

Romans 5:12
12 Therefore, as through one man sin entered into the world, and death through sin; and so death passed unto all men, for that all sinned.

1 Corinthians 11:29-30
29 For he that eateth and drinketh, eateth and drinketh judgment unto himself, if he discern not the body.
30 For this cause many among you are weak and sickly, and not a few sleep.

James 1:15
15 Then the lust, when it hath conceived, beareth sin: and the sin, when it is fullgrown, bringeth forth death.

James 5:5
5 Ye have lived delicately on the earth, and taken your pleasure; ye have nourished your hearts in a day of slaughter.

Hopelessness, Hope, and Depression

Hopelessness seems to take all of the energy from our lives. It fuels negative thoughts that pull us down even more. Our will to move our life forward is damaged. Jesus is our hope, but do we just logically or intuitively know it? Or do we experientially know that Jesus is our hope by living with Him daily? Of course, living a life of hope is what we want to achieve.

Perhaps you have experienced an event in your life where you felt completely hopeless. Jesus wasn't in your life then, or so you thought. You hadn't knocked on His door yet, or you may have been too young and at the mercy of others. Jesus knows your situation; He was there from the beginning, He is here with you now, and He will be there at the end. Ask Jesus to replace hopelessness with hope in your life.

> *Medical science has found a connection between hopelessness and depression, and I have confirmed that link through my discussions.*

Medical science has also found a connection between hopelessness and depression, and I have confirmed that link through my discussions. People I asked who have suffered from depression all said they had feelings of hopelessness while they were depressed.

Remember!
When praying scripture, give Jesus permission to search for lies and unbelief and replace them with God's truth.

Romans 15:13-14   Key Verse
13 Now the God of hope fill you with all joy and peace in believing, that ye may abound in hope, in the power of the Holy Spirit.
14 And I myself also am persuaded of you, my brethren, that ye yourselves are full of goodness, filled with all knowledge, able also to admonish one another.

Psalms 42:11   Key Verse
11 Why art thou cast down, O my soul? And why art thou disquieted within me? Hope thou in God; For I shall yet praise him, Who is the help of my countenance, and my God.

1 Peter 1:21   Key Verse
21 who through him are believers in God, that raised him from the dead, and gave him glory; so that your faith and hope might be in God.

Proverbs 13:12   Key Verse
12 Hope deferred maketh the heart sick; But when the desire cometh, it is a tree of life.

Joshua 23:14

14 And, behold, this day I am going the way of all the earth: and ye know in all your hearts and in all your souls, that not one thing hath failed of all the good things which Jehovah your God spake concerning you; all are come to pass unto you, not one thing hath failed thereof.

Psalms 33:16-18

16 There is no king saved by the multitude of a host: A mighty man is not delivered by great strength.

17 A horse is a vain thing for safety; Neither doth he deliver any by his great power.

18 Behold, the eye of Jehovah is upon them that fear him, Upon them that hope in his lovingkindness;

Psalms 34:18-22

18 Jehovah is nigh unto them that are of a broken heart, And saveth such as are of a contrite spirit.

19 Many are the afflictions of the righteous; But Jehovah delivereth him out of them all.

20 He keepeth all his bones: Not one of them is broken.

21 Evil shall slay the wicked; And they that hate the righteous shall be condemned.

22 Jehovah redeemeth the soul of his servants; And none of them that take refuge in him shall be condemned.

Psalms 71:5

5 For thou art my hope, O Lord Jehovah: Thou art my trust from my youth.

Psalms 130:7

7 O Israel, hope in Jehovah; For with Jehovah there is lovingkindness, And with him is plenteous redempti

Isaiah 29:14

14 therefore, behold, I will proceed to do a marvellous work among

this people, even a marvellous work and a wonder; and the wisdom of their wise men shall perish, and the understanding of their prudent men shall be hid.
on.
Lord, I am oppressed, be thou my surety.

Isaiah 38:14

14 Like a swallow or a crane, so did I chatter; I did moan as a dove; mine eyes fail with looking upward: O Psalms 16:9
9 Therefore my heart is glad, and my glory rejoiceth; My flesh also shall dwell in safety.

Jeremiah 18:12

12 But they say, It is in vain; for we will walk after our own devices, and we will do every one after the stubbornness of his evil heart.

Jeremiah 29:11-12

11 For I know the thoughts that I think toward you, saith Jehovah, thoughts of peace, and not of evil, to give you hope in your latter end.
12 And ye shall call upon me, and ye shall go and pray unto me, and I will hearken unto you.

Ezekiel 37:14

14 And I will put my Spirit in you, and ye shall live, and I will place you in your own land: and ye shall know that I, Jehovah, have spoken it and performed it, saith Jehovah.

John 3:17

17 For God sent not the Son into the world to judge the world; but that the world should be saved through him.

John 8:32

32 and ye shall know the truth, and the truth shall make you free.

John 14:1-4

1 Let not your heart be troubled: believe in God, believe also in me.
2 In my Father's house are many mansions; if it were not so, I would have told you; for I go to prepare a place for you.
3 And if I go and prepare a place for you, I come again, and will receive you unto myself; that where I am, there ye may be also.
4 And whither I go, ye know the way.

John 9:31 (ASV)

31 We know that God heareth not sinners: but if any man be a worshipper of God, and do his will, him he heareth.

Romans 5:6-7

6 For while we were yet weak, in due season Christ died for the ungodly.
7 For scarcely for a righteous man will one die: for peradventure for the good man some one would even dare to die.

Romans 6:4-8

4 We were buried therefore with him through baptism unto death: that like as Christ was raised from the dead through the glory of the Father, so we also might walk in newness of life.
5 For if we have become united with him in the likeness of his death, we shall be also in the likeness of his resurrection;
6 knowing this, that our old man was crucified with him, that the body of sin might be done away, that so we should no longer be in bondage to sin;
7 for he that hath died is justified from sin.
8 But if we died with Christ, we believe that we shall also live with him;

Galatians 5:22-23

22 But the fruit of the Spirit is love, joy, peace, longsuffering, kindness, goodness, faithfulness,
23 meekness, self-control; against such there is no law.

Galatians 6:14

14 But far be it from me to glory, save in the cross of our Lord Jesus Christ, through which the world hath been crucified unto me, and I unto the world.

Ephesians 1:18

18 having the eyes of your heart enlightened, that ye may know what is the hope of his calling, what the riches of the glory of his inheritance in the saints,

Ephesians 2:2

2 wherein ye once walked according to the course of this world, according to the prince of the powers of the air, of the spirit that now worketh in the sons of disobedience;

Philippians 1:6

6 being confident of this very thing, that he who began a good work in you will perfect it until the day of Jesus Christ:

Colossians 1:5

5 because of the hope which is laid up for you in the heavens, whereof ye heard before in the word of the truth of the gospel,

Colossians 1:27

27 to whom God was pleased to make known what is the riches of the glory of this mystery among the Gentiles, which is Christ in you, the hope of glory:

Colossians 1:29

29 whereunto I labor also, striving according to his working, which worketh in me mightily.

Colossians 2:2-5

2 that their hearts may be comforted, they being knit together in love, and unto all riches of the full assurance of understanding, that they may know the mystery of God, even Christ,

3 in whom are all the treasures of wisdom and knowledge hidden.
4 This I say, that no one may delude you with persuasiveness of speech.
5 For though I am absent in the flesh, yet am I with you in the spirit, joying and beholding your order, and the stedfastness of your faith in Christ.

Hebrews 6:19
19 which we have as an anchor of the soul, a hope both sure and stedfast and entering into that which is within the veil;

Hebrews 10:23
23 let us hold fast the confession of our hope that it waver not; for he is faithful that promised:

Hebrews 12:28
28 Wherefore, receiving a kingdom that cannot be shaken, let us have grace, whereby we may offer service well-pleasing to God with reverence and awe:

1 Peter 1:3-4
3 Blessed be the God and Father of our Lord Jesus Christ, who according to his great mercy begat us again unto a living hope by the resurrection of Jesus Christ from the dead,
4 unto an inheritance incorruptible, and undefiled, and that fadeth not away, reserved in heaven for you,

1 Peter 1:13
13 Wherefore girding up the loins of your mind, be sober and set your hope perfectly on the grace that is to be brought unto you at the revelation of Jesus Christ;

1 Peter 2:9-10
9 But ye are a elect race, a royal priesthood, a holy nation, a people for God's own possession, that ye may show forth the excellencies of him who called you out of darkness into his marvellous light:

10 who in time past were no people, but now are the people of God: who had not obtained mercy, but now have obtained mercy.

1 John 3:3
3 And every one that hath this hope set on him purifieth himself, even as he is pure.

INIQUITY

You may have vowed not to repeat the not-so-nice and sinful things your parents did, yet find that you are doing the same thing, and/or have great fear of being like them. We are not responsible for the sins of our parents, but we may be under a generational curse—the consequences of the sins of our family lineage. We need to break free of these negative strongholds on our life, those caused by our own choices and those caused by the sins of our predecessors.

> *Praise God that He is stronger than any of our battles!*

It is sometimes difficult to escape these strongholds because they may be reinforced through our own habits of sin or through many generations within our family. Praise God that He is stronger than any of our battles! You must call on Jesus and your helper, the Holy Spirit, for the strength and ability to overcome sin and the effects of generational curses. Jesus took away the sins of the world for all those who believe with true repentance toward God. The Word of God promises generational blessings—not curses—for your obedience and faith!

Remember!
When praying scripture, give Jesus permission to search for lies and unbelief and replace them with God's truth.

Psalms 119:133   Key Verse
133 Establish my footsteps in thy word; And let not any iniquity have dominion over me.

Isaiah 6:7   Key Verse
7 and he touched my mouth with it, and said, Lo, this hath touched thy lips; and thine iniquity is taken away, and thy sin forgiven.

Deuteronomy 5:7-9
7 Thou shalt have no other gods before me.
8 Thou shalt not make unto thee a graven image, nor any likeness of anything that is in heaven above, or that is in the earth beneath, or that is in the water under the earth:
9 thou shalt not bow down thyself unto them, nor serve them; for I, Jehovah, thy God, am a jealous God, visiting the iniquity of the fathers upon the children, and upon the third and upon the fourth generation of them that hate me;

Proverbs 12:7
7 The wicked are overthrown, and are not; But the house of the righteous shall stand.

Proverbs 17:13
13 Whoso rewardeth evil for good, Evil shall not depart from his house.

Proverbs 27:7
7 The full soul loatheth a honeycomb; But to the hungry soul every bitter thing is sweet.

Isaiah 53:11
11 He shall see of the travail of his soul, and shall be satisfied: by the knowledge of himself shall my righteous servant justify many; and he shall bear their iniquities.

Jeremiah 31:29
29 In those days they shall say no more, The fathers have eaten sour grapes, and the children's teeth are set on edge.

Jeremiah 31:34
34 and they shall teach no more every man his neighbor, and every man his brother, saying, Know Jehovah; for they shall all know me, from the least of them unto the greatest of them, saith Jehovah: for I will forgive their iniquity, and their sin will I remember no more.

Ezekiel 18:20
20 The soul that sinneth, it shall die: the son shall not bear the iniquity of the father, neither shall the father bear the iniquity of the son; the righteousness of the righteous shall be upon him, and the wickedness of the wicked shall be upon him.

Luke 13:27
27 and he shall say, I tell you, I know not whence ye are; depart from me, all ye workers of iniquity.

Joy and Mental Stability

God does not want us to be depressed, lethargic, pessimistic, or wallowing in self-pity. He wants our life to be filled with joy. Our mental stability is dependent, to a great extent, on what we choose to think about throughout the day and our self-talk. Because our mind is like a storage container, we must guard what enters into it to avoid problems. We must control what we do with our senses. Our eyes, for example, bring us visual images, some of which are good and some not so good. Sounds, smells, and touches can also be uplifting or provide negative temptations and opportunities for sin.

Thousands of thoughts go through our mind each day. Most thoughts are our own, but some are not. Satan and the things of this fallen world have the ability to influence our thoughts if we let them. We can be tempted and then condemned. Satan seems to work hard to try and remind us

> *Satan and the things of this fallen world have the ability to influence our thoughts if we let them.*

about all those negative memories. It can become spiritual warfare if you allow it. However, you have the authority through Jesus Christ, to take your thoughts captive, to discern the source of such negativity, and determine to focus on Godly, virtuous thoughts, not lies and temptations.

God speaks to us quietly. If we allow Satan to scream negativity into our mind, we will have a hard time hearing God's voice. So we must prepare our mind to hear God by cleaning house and guarding what goes in. We can clean our mind by seeking healing for our wounds, seeking forgiveness for our sins, and forgiving those who have sinned against us. Our self-talk should become uplifting and motivational as we meditate on the beautiful things of God, His Word, His Will, and His Wisdom.

Our brain controls our bodily functions. All bodily functions cease when our brain is dead. So it makes sense that when our mind/brain is out of balance, we may have body chemicals out of balance. These chemicals affect our digestive system, our energy, our immune system, our mood, and more. The subject of joy and our mental state is not a stand-alone topic; it affects many other topics which are discussed in this book.

Remember!
When praying scripture, give Jesus permission to search for lies and unbelief and replace them with God's truth.

Romans 14:17 Key Verse
17 for the kingdom of God is not eating and drinking, but righteousness and peace and joy in the Holy Spirit.

Joy and Mental Stability

Psalms 118:24   Key Verse
24 This is the day which Jehovah hath made; We will rejoice and be glad in it.

Nehemiah 8:10
10 Then he said unto them, Go your way, eat the fat, and drink the sweet, and send portions unto him for whom nothing is prepared; for this day is holy unto our Lord: neither be ye grieved; for the joy of Jehovah is your strength.

Psalms 94:19
19 In the multitude of my thoughts within me Thy comforts delight my soul.

Proverbs 15:13
13 A glad heart maketh a cheerful countenance; But by sorrow of heart the spirit is broken.

Proverbs 15:15
15 All the days of the afflicted are evil; But he that is of a cheerful heart hath a continual feast.

Jeremiah 15:16
16 Thy words were found, and I did eat them; and thy words were unto me a joy and the rejoicing of my heart: for I am called by thy name, O Jehovah, God of hosts.

Zephaniah 3:17
17 Jehovah thy God is in the midst of thee, a mighty one who will save; he will rejoice over thee with joy; he will rest in his love; he will joy over thee with singing.

Luke 1:47
47 And my spirit hath rejoiced in God my Saviour.
Proverbs 29:18 (ASV)
18 Where there is no vision, the people cast off restraint; But he that

keepeth the law, happy is he.

John 15:11
11 These things have I spoken unto you, that my joy may be in you, and that your joy may be made full.
Colossians 1:11 (ASV)
11 strengthened with all power, according to the might of his glory, unto all patience and longsuffering with joy;

John 16:24
24 Hitherto have ye asked nothing in my name: ask, and ye shall receive, that your joy may be made full.
James 1:8 (ASV)
8 a doubleminded man, unstable in all his ways.

John 17:13
13 But now I come to thee; and these things I speak in the world, that they may have my joy made full in themselves.

Philippians 4:4
4 Rejoice in the Lord always: again I will say, Rejoice.

2 Timothy 1:7
7 For God gave us not a spirit of fearfulness; but of power and love and discipline.

James 1:2
2 Count it all joy, my brethren, when ye fall into manifold temptations;

1 Peter 1:8
8 whom not having seen ye love; on whom, though now ye see him not, yet believing, ye rejoice greatly with joy unspeakable and full of glory:

Loneliness and Feeling Forsaken

Loneliness is that feeling of having a hole in your heart, where life's fullness seems to have leaked out. Humans were not created to be an island unto themselves. Although loneliness may appear benign, it is not. Satan can use our feelings of loneliness to draw us to destructive people and activities. And people can feel alone and empty even with people around them. We have seen examples of this when famous people succumb to suicide.

Maybe we are feeling lonely because we are living out what we believe is true about ourselves. If a person had been abandoned sometime earlier in their life, it is possible they currently identify with that abandoned person of the past. With so many children being raised in single-parent families, it is no wonder so many have feelings of abandonment. The reasons for these situations are not as important as our current perception. There

> *Maybe we are feeling lonely because we are living out what we believe is true about ourselves.*

may be distortions and lies in our perception of past events. Satan uses lies to tempt us. Many give in to that temptation and attempt to wrongly fill their empty heart.

Others have constructed a protective wall around themselves. They have been hurt in the past and have vowed not to let it happen again. Once they have dug in their heels and proclaimed their stand to the spirit world, they find it difficult to change. In effect, they have allowed one stronghold to keep them submitted to another. It's like putting two combination locks on a door, only two people each know one combination, and they are not cooperating with each other.

As you let Jesus into more of your life and you gain freedom, feelings of loneliness will diminish. Jesus is the companion everyone needs.

Remember!
When praying scripture, give Jesus permission to search for lies and unbelief and replace them with God's truth.

John 16:32   Key Verse
32 Behold, the hour cometh, yea, is come, that ye shall be scattered, every man to his own, and shall leave me alone: and yet I am not alone, because the Father is with me.

John 14:18   Key Verse
18 I will not leave you desolate: I come unto you.

Deuteronomy 31:6   Key Verse
6 Be strong and of good courage, fear not, nor be affrighted at them: for Jehovah thy God, he it is that doth go with thee; he will not fail thee, nor forsake thee.

Genesis 28:15

15 And, behold, I am with thee, and will keep thee, whithersoever thou goest, and will bring thee again into this land. For I will not leave thee, until I have done that which I have spoken to thee of.

Joshua 1:5

5 There shall not any man be able to stand before thee all the days of thy life. as I was with Moses, so I will be with thee; I will not fail thee, nor forsake thee.

1 Kings 6:13

13 And I will dwell among the children of Israel, and will not forsake my people Israel.

Psalms 9:9

9 Jehovah also will be a high tower for the oppressed, A high tower in times of trouble;

Psalms 25:16

16 Turn thee unto me, and have mercy upon me; For I am desolate and afflicted.

Psalms 27:9-10

9 Hide not thy face from me; Put not thy servant away in anger: Thou hast been my help; Cast me not off, neither forsake me, O God of my salvation.
10 When my father and my mother forsake me, Then Jehovah will take me up.

Psalms 40:10-11

10 I have not hid thy righteousness within my heart; I have declared thy faithfulness and thy salvation; I have not concealed thy lovingkindness and thy truth from the great assembly.
11 Withhold not thou thy tender mercies from me, O Jehovah; Let thy lovingkindness and thy truth continually preserve me.

Psalms 40:17
17 But I am poor and needy; Yet the Lord thinketh upon me: Thou art my help and my deliverer; Make no tarrying, O my God.

Isaiah 49:15
15 Can a woman forget her sucking child, that she should not have compassion on the son of her womb? yea, these may forget, yet will not I forget thee.

Isaiah 58:9
9 Then shalt thou call, and Jehovah will answer; thou shalt cry, and he will say, Here I am. If thou take away from the midst of thee the yoke, the putting forth of the finger, and speaking wickedly;

Matthew 10:32
32 Every one therefore who shall confess me before men, him will I also confess before my Father who is in heaven.

Matthew 28:20
20 teaching them to observe all things whatsoever I commanded you: and lo, I am with you always, even unto the end of the world

Colossians 2:10
10 and in him ye are made full, who is the head of all principality and power:

Hebrews 13:5
5 Be ye free from the love of money; content with such things as ye have: for himself hath said, I will in no wise fail thee, neither will I in any wise forsake thee.

James 4:8
8 Draw nigh to God, and he will draw nigh to you. Cleanse your hands, ye sinners; and purify your hearts, ye doubleminded.

LOVE

The following scripture verses speak better about love than any description I could have written.

1 Corinthians 13:1-7
1 If I speak with the tongues of men and of angels, but have not love, I am become sounding brass, or a clanging cymbal. 2 And if I have the gift of prophecy, and know all mysteries and all knowledge; and if I have all faith, so as to remove mountains, but have not love, I am nothing.
3 And if I bestow all my goods to feed the poor, and if I give my body to be burned, but have not love, it profiteth me nothing. 4 Love suffereth long, and is kind; love envieth not; love vaunteth not itself, is not puffed up, 5 doth not behave itself unseemly, seeketh not its own, is not provoked, taketh not account of evil; 6 rejoiceth not in unrighteousness, but rejoiceth with the truth;
7 beareth all things, believeth all things, hopeth all things, endureth all things.

> *Knowing God's definition of love can help us live a Spirit-led life according to His truth.*

God created us with the inherent need for love. Love is a multibillion dollar industry, of which Valentine's Day is one example. But what is love? Some define love as a feeling, but the problem with feelings is that they are like the weather and can change quickly. Feelings are influenced by our moods, signs, appetites, and the rest of our sensory receptors. Feelings can also be influenced by our memories, which can contain wounds or joys from our past. This can make relying on feelings deceptive at best. Knowing instead God's definition of love can help us live a Spirit-led life according to His truth. And of course it goes without saying, Jesus is love.

Remember!
When praying scripture, give Jesus permission to search for lies and unbelief and replace them with God's truth.

1 John 4:9-10   Key Verse
9 Herein was the love of God manifested in us, that God hath sent his only begotten Son into the world that we might live through him.
10 Herein is love, not that we loved God, but that he loved us, and sent his Son to be the propitiation for our sins.

1 Thessalonians 4:9   Key Verse
9 But concerning love of the brethren ye have no need that one write unto you: for ye yourselves are taught of God to love one another;

Deuteronomy 6:5   Key Verse
5 and thou shalt love Jehovah thy God with all thy heart, and with

all thy soul, and with all thy might.

Deuteronomy 7:13
13 and he will love thee, and bless thee, and multiply thee; he will also bless the fruit of thy body and the fruit of thy ground, thy grain and thy new wine and thine oil, the increase of thy cattle and the young of thy flock, in the land which he sware unto thy fathers to give thee.

1 Kings 10:9
9 Blessed be Jehovah thy God, who delighted in thee, to set thee on the throne of Israel: because Jehovah loved Israel for ever, therefore made he thee king, to do justice and righteousness.

Psalms 91:14
14 Because he hath set his love upon me, therefore will I deliver him: I will set him on high, because he hath known my name.

Psalms 142:4
4 Look on my right hand, and see; For there is no man that knoweth me: Refuge hath failed me; No man careth for my soul.

Proverbs 15:17
17 Better is a dinner of herbs, where love is, Than a stalled ox and hatred therewith.

Proverbs 18:20-21
20 A man's belly shall be filled with the fruit of his mouth; With the increase of his lips shall he be satisfied.
21 Death and life are in the power of the tongue; And they that love it shall eat the fruit thereof.

Song of Songs 8:6
6 Set me as a seal upon thy heart, As a seal upon thine arm: For love is strong as death; Jealousy is cruel as Sheol; The flashes thereof are flashes of fire, A very flame of Jehovah.

Jeremiah 31:3

3 Jehovah appeared of old unto me, saying, Yea, I have loved thee with an everlasting love: therefore with lovingkindness have I drawn thee.

Ezekiel 16:8

8 Now when I passed by thee, and looked upon thee, behold, thy time was the time of love; and I spread my skirt over thee, and covered thy nakedness: yea, I sware unto thee, and entered into a covenant with thee, saith the Lord Jehovah, and thou becamest mine.

Hosea 14:4

4 I will heal their backsliding, I will love them freely; for mine anger is turned away from him.

Proverbs 15:9 (ASV)

9 The way of the wicked is an abomination to Jehovah; But he loveth him that followeth after righteousness.

Zephaniah 3:17

17 Jehovah thy God is in the midst of thee, a mighty one who will save; he will rejoice over thee with joy; he will rest in his love; he will joy over thee with singing.

John 3:16

16 For God so loved the world, that he gave his only begotten Son, that whosoever believeth on him should not perish, but have eternal life.

John 13:34 (Hatefulness)

34 A new commandment I give unto you, that ye love one another; even as I have loved you, that ye also love one another.

John 15:9

9 Even as the Father hath loved me, I also have loved you: abide ye in my love.

John 16:27

27 for the Father himself loveth you, because ye have loved me, and have believed that I came forth from the Father.

John 17:23

23 I in them, and thou in me, that they may be perfected into one; that the world may know that thou didst send me, and lovedst them, even as thou lovedst me.

Romans 1:7

7 To all that are in Rome, beloved of God, called to be saints: Grace to you and peace from God our Father and the Lord Jesus Christ.

Romans 5:5

5 and hope putteth not to shame; because the love of God hath been shed abroad in our hearts through the Holy Spirit which was given unto us.

Romans 8:38-39

38 For I am persuaded, that neither death, nor life, nor angels, nor principalities, nor things present, nor things to come, nor powers, 39 nor height, nor depth, nor any other creature, shall be able to separate us from the love of God, which is in Christ Jesus our Lord.

Romans 12:9

9 Let love be without hypocrisy. Abhor that which is evil; cleave to that which is good.

Galatians 2:20

20 I have been crucified with Christ; and it is no longer I that live, but Christ living in me: and that life which I now live in the flesh I live in faith, the faith which is in the Son of God, who loved me, and gave himself up for me.

Ephesians 1:3

3 Blessed be the God and Father of our Lord Jesus Christ, who hath blessed us with every spiritual blessing in the heavenly places in Christ:

Ephesians 2:4-7

4 but God, being rich in mercy, for his great love wherewith he loved us,
5 even when we were dead through our trespasses, made us alive together with Christ (by grace have ye been saved),
6 and raised us up with him, and made us to sit with him in the heavenly places, in Christ Jesus:
7 that in the ages to come he might show the exceeding riches of his grace in kindness toward us in Christ Jesus:

Ephesians 3:14-21

14 For this cause I bow my knees unto the Father,
15 from whom every family in heaven and on earth is named,
16 that he would grant you, according to the riches of his glory, that ye may be strengthened with power through his Spirit in the inward man;
17 that Christ may dwell in your hearts through faith; to the end that ye, being rooted and grounded in love,
18 may be strong to apprehend with all the saints what is the breadth and length and height and depth,
19 and to know the love of Christ which passeth knowledge, that ye may be filled unto all the fulness of God.
20 Now unto him that is able to do exceeding abundantly above all that we ask or think, according to the power that worketh in us,
21 unto him be the glory in the church and in Christ Jesus unto all generations for ever and ever. Amen.

Colossians 1:12-14

12 giving thanks unto the Father, who made us meet to be partakers of the inheritance of the saints in light;
13 who delivered us out of the power of darkness, and translated us into the kingdom of the Son of his love;
14 in whom we have our redemption, the forgiveness of our sins:

Colossians 3:14-15

14 and above all these things put on love, which is the bond of perfectness.
15 And let the peace of Christ rule in your hearts, to the which also ye were called in one body; and be ye thankful.

1 John 3:1

1 Behold what manner of love the Father hath bestowed upon us, that we should be called children of God; and such we are. For this cause the world knoweth us not, because it knew him not.

1 John 3:14

14 We know that we have passed out of death into life, because we love the brethren. He that loveth not abideth in death.

1 John 4:16-20

16 And we know and have believed the love which God hath in us. God is love; and he that abideth in love abideth in God, and God abideth in him.
17 Herein is love made perfect with us, that we may have boldness in the day of judgment; because as he is, even so are we in this world.
18 There is no fear in love: but perfect love casteth out fear, because fear hath punishment; and he that feareth is not made perfect in love.
19 We love, because he first loved us.
20 If a man say, I love God, and hateth his brother, he is a liar: for he that loveth not his brother whom he hath seen, cannot love God whom he hath not seen.

2 John 1:3

3 Grace, mercy, peace shall be with us, from God the Father, and from Jesus Christ, the Son of the Father, in truth and love.

If you don't love God, your ability to receive love, or loving yourself or your neighbor may be distorted. The following scripture verses are about loving God.

Proverbs 16:13
13 Righteous lips are the delight of kings; And they love him that speaketh right.

Matthew 22:37
37 And he said unto him, Thou shalt love the Lord thy God with all thy heart, and with all thy soul, and with all thy mind.

John 14:21-24
21 He that hath my commandments, and keepeth them, he it is that loveth me: and he that loveth me shall be loved of my Father, and I will love him, and will manifest myself unto him.
22 Judas (not Iscariot) saith unto him, Lord, what is come to pass that thou wilt manifest thyself unto us, and not unto the world?
23 Jesus answered and said unto him, If a man love me, he will keep my word: and my Father will love him, and we will come unto him, and make our abode with him.
24 He that loveth me not keepeth not my words: and the word which ye hear is not mine, but the Father's who sent me.

John 14:31
31 but that the world may know that I love the Father, and as the Father gave me commandment, even so I do.

2 John 1:6
6 And this is love, that we should walk after his commandments. This is the commandment, even as ye heard from the beginning, that ye should walk in it.

Lust and Covetousness

Lust is an inordinate desire or craving for the pleasure of worldly things. This is based on a distorted perception of who we are in the world. We can never find true satisfaction in fulfilling these desires according to the ways of the world, which is fallen. In fact, the farther we go down this road of lust and covetousness, the more distant satisfaction becomes. Reality becomes obscure and we make decisions based on the feelings and longings we want fulfilled. The decisions we make lead to more problems in our life and the downward spiral continues. Behind the scenes, Satan is cheering us on.

> *We can never find true satisfaction in fulfilling these desires according to the ways of the world, which is fallen.*

We are all tempted at times, and many people fall into addictions, such as pornography. While there may be a number of reasons some of us have greater problems with lust, I believe that present unmet needs and unmet needs of the past may influence a person to choose deviant behavior. A child's perception of events may not be true reality, nevertheless, their belief about who they think they are becomes burned into their memory, which affects how they live today.

For example, people try to fill their unmet needs for love through sexual encounters. But the thrill soon wears off and is never fulfilling over the long haul. Only Jesus can fill the need for love—past, present, and future. This is especially important to understand if our family members have given us the short end of the stick. Another example of people trying to meet unfulfilled needs is when they think they need the latest, best-looking, high-status material things. This can lead to financial disaster. Only Jesus can verify who we are and help us to overcome the fears of what other people think of us and teach us that following His plan for our lives is all that really matters.

Let Jesus, with the power of the Word, help you overcome the temptations of lust and covetousness. As with many other negative strongholds, the foundational roots of lust and covetousness overlap those of other topics. For instance, coveting something someone else has likely shows a lack of contentment and possibly a weak self-worth. Don't hesitate to ask the Holy Spirit to help you resist temptations while you work out those roots. Seek to replace that longing pressure, those desires, with God's peace. His peace and contentment will bring you purpose and fulfillment.

Remember!
When praying scripture, give Jesus permission to search for lies and unbelief and replace them with God's truth.

Galatians 5:16   Key Verse
16 But I say, walk by the Spirit, and ye shall not fulfil the lust of the flesh.

Colossians 3:5   Key Verse
5 Put to death therefore your members which are upon the earth: fornication, uncleanness, passion, evil desire, and covetousness, which is idolatry;

Exodus 20:17   Key Verse
17 Thou shalt not covet thy neighbor's house, thou shalt not covet thy neighbor's wife, nor his man-servant, nor his maid-servant, nor his ox, nor his ass, nor anything that is thy neighbor's.

Job 31:25
25 If I have rejoiced because my wealth was great, And because my hand had gotten much;

Proverbs 6:25
25 Lust not after her beauty in thy heart; Neither let her take thee with her eyelids.

Proverbs 11:24
24 There is that scattereth, and increaseth yet more; And there is that withholdeth more than is meet, but it tendeth only to want.

Proverbs 21:26
26 There is that coveteth greedily all the day long; But the righteous giveth and withholdeth not.

Ecclesiastes 5:10
10 He that loveth silver shall not be satisfied with silver; nor he that loveth abundance, with increase: this also is vanity.

Hosea 4:11
11 Whoredom and wine and new wine take away the understanding.

Matthew 6:20

20 but lay up for yourselves treasures in heaven, where neither moth nor rust doth consume, and where thieves do not break through nor steal:

Matthew 6:24-25

24 No man can serve two masters; for either he will hate the one, and love the other; or else he will hold to one, and despise the other. Ye cannot serve God and mammon.
25 Therefore I say unto you, be not anxious for your life, what ye shall eat, or what ye shall drink; nor yet for your body, what ye shall put on. Is not the life more than the food, and the body than the raiment?

Mark 4:19

19 and the cares of the world, and the deceitfulness of riches, and the lusts of other things entering in, choke the word, and it becometh unfruitful.

Romans 1:21

21 because that, knowing God, they glorified him not as God, neither gave thanks; but became vain in their reasonings, and their senseless heart was darkened.

Romans 1:27

27 and likewise also the men, leaving the natural use of the woman, burned in their lust one toward another, men with men working unseemliness, and receiving in themselves that recompense of their error which was due.

Romans 13:14

14 But put ye on the Lord Jesus Christ, and make not provision for the flesh, to fulfil the lusts thereof.

Ephesians 4:22

22 that ye put away, as concerning your former manner of life, the old man, that waxeth corrupt after the lusts of deceit;

Ephesians 5:3-5
3 But fornication, and all uncleanness, or covetousness, let it not even be named among you, as becometh saints;
4 nor filthiness, nor foolish talking, or jesting, which are not befitting: but rather giving of thanks.
5 For this ye know of a surety, that no fornicator, nor unclean person, nor covetous man, who is an idolater, hath any inheritance in the kingdom of Christ and God.

Philippians 3:19
19 whose end is perdition, whose god is the belly, and whose glory is in their shame, who mind earthly things.

Jude 1:11 (ASV)
11 Woe unto them! For they went in the way of Cain, and ran riotously in the error of Balaam for hire, and perished in the gainsaying of Korah.

1 Thessalonians 4:3-5
3 For this is the will of God, even your sanctification, that ye abstain from fornication;
4 that each one of you know how to possess himself of his own vessel in sanctification and honor,
5 not in the passion of lust, even as the Gentiles who know not God;

1 Timothy 6:9
9 But they that are minded to be rich fall into a temptation and a snare and many foolish and hurtful lusts, such as drown men in destruction and perdition.

2 Timothy 2:22
22 after righteousness, faith, love, pace, with them that call on the Lord out of a pure heart.

Titus 2:12

12 instructing us, to the intent that, denying ungodliness and worldly lusts, we should live soberly and righteously and godly in this present world;

James 1:14-15

14 but each man is tempted, when he is drawn away by his own lust, and enticed.
15 Then the lust, when it hath conceived, beareth sin: and the sin, when it is fullgrown, bringeth forth death.

James 4:1-3

1 Whence come wars and whence come fightings among you? come they not hence, even of your pleasures that war in your members?
2 Ye lust, and have not: ye kill, and covet, and cannot obtain: ye fight and war; ye have not, because ye ask not.
3 Ye ask, and receive not, because ye ask amiss, that ye may spend it in your pleasures.

1 John 2:15-17

15 Love not the world, neither the things that are in the world. If any man love the world, the love of the Father is not in him.
16 For all that is in the world, the lust of the flesh and the lust of the eyes and the vain glory of life, is not of the Father, but is of the world.
17 And the world passeth away, and the lust thereof: but he that doeth the will of God abideth for ever.

Obedience, Rebellion, and God's Will & Protection

Have you even known a very rebellious child and were able to observe them into adulthood? If they are constantly in trouble or in crisis, you can be sure their life is marked with rebellion. It is like a rudderless ship that is totally at the mercy of the wind and currents. Events control these people and they are unable to break out of their prison. Their lives are going nowhere.

Obedience gives us freedom in our lives. If you find yourself always working hard, like paddling upstream but getting nowhere, consider that this area of your life needs to be revitalized. Jesus said, "My yoke is easy." So if you are tired out, think about placing your life under God's control. Many scripture verses are "if/then," which means "if" we do such and such, "then" God will respond accordingly.

> **Obedience gives us freedom in our lives.**

We tend to focus on the "then," which are the good things we desire from God. However, many of God's promises are conditional, they depend upon our obedience. Let these scripture verses help you. Allow God to reveal to you His truths about following Him.

Remember!
When praying scripture, give Jesus permission to search for lies and unbelief and replace them with God's truth.

2 Corinthians 10:18   Key Verse
18 For not he that commendeth himself is approved, but whom the Lord commendeth.

Ephesians 6:2   Key Verse
2 Honor thy father and mother (which is the first commandment with promise),

Hebrews 13:17   Key Verse
17 Obey them that have the rule over you, and submit to them: for they watch in behalf of your souls, as they that shall give account; that they may do this with joy, and not with grief: for this were unprofitable for you.

John 15:14   Key Verse
14 Ye are my friends, if ye do the things which I command you.

Genesis 2:16-17
16 And Jehovah God commanded the man, saying, Of every tree of the garden thou mayest freely eat:
17 but of the tree of the knowledge of good and evil, thou shalt not eat of it: for in the day that thou eatest thereof thou shalt surely die.

Exodus 6:6-7

6 Wherefore say unto the children of Israel, I am Jehovah, and I will bring you out from under the burdens of the Egyptians, and I will rid you out of their bondage, and I will redeem you with an outstretched arm, and with great judgments:
7 and I will take you to me for a people, and I will be to you a God; and ye shall know that I am Jehovah your God, who bringeth you out from under the burdens of the Egyptians.

Exodus 20:20

20 And Moses said unto the people, Fear not: for God is come to prove you, and that his fear may be before you, that ye sin not.

Deuteronomy 27:16

16 Cursed be he that setteth light by his father or his mother. And all the people shall say, Amen.

1 Samuel 15:22-23

22 And Samuel said, Hath Jehovah as great delight in burnt-offerings and sacrifices, as in obeying the voice of Jehovah? Behold, to obey is better than sacrifice, and to hearken than the fat of rams.
23 For rebellion is as the sin of witchcraft, and stubbornness is as idolatry and teraphim. Because thou hast rejected the word of Jehovah, he hath also rejected thee from being king.

1 Chronicles 28:9

9 And thou, Solomon my son, know thou the God of thy father, and serve him with a perfect heart and with a willing mind; for Jehovah searcheth all hearts, and understandeth all the imaginations of the thoughts: if thou seek him, he will be found of thee; but if thou forsake him, he will cast thee off for ever.

Job 8:5-6

5 If thou wouldest seek diligently unto God, And make thy supplication to the Almighty;
6 If thou wert pure and upright: Surely now he would awake for

thee, And make the habitation of thy righteousness prosperous.

Psalms 8:6

6 Thou makest him to have dominion over the works of thy hands; Thou hast put all things under his feet:

Psalms 32:6

6 For this let every one that is godly pray unto thee in a time when thou mayest be found: Surely when the great waters overflow they shall not reach unto him.

Psalms 40:7-8

7 Then said I, Lo, I am come; In the roll of the book it is written of me:
8 I delight to do thy will, O my God; Yea, thy law is within my heart.

Psalms 51:16-17

16 For thou delightest not in sacrifice; Else would I give it: Thou hast no pleasure in burnt-offering.
17 The sacrifices of God are a broken spirit: A broken and contrite heart, O God, thou wilt not despise.

Psalms 91:1-2

1 He that dwelleth in the secret place of the Most High shall abide under the shadow of the Almighty.
2 I will say of Jehovah, He is my refuge and my fortress; My God, in whom I trust.

Psalms 119:67

67 Before I was afflicted I went astray; But now I observe thy word.

Psalms 119:75

75 I know, O Jehovah, that thy judgments are righteous, And that in faithfulness thou hast afflicted me.

Ecclesiastes 12:13
13 This is the end of the matter; all hath been heard: fear God, and keep his commandments; for this is the whole duty of man.
James 1:22 (ASV)
22 But be ye doers of the word, and not hearers only, deluding your own selves.

Isaiah 28:12
12 to whom he said, This is the rest, give ye rest to him that is weary; and this is the refreshing: yet they would not hear.

Isaiah 43:2
2 When thou passest through the waters, I will be with thee; and through the rivers, they shall not overflow thee: when thou walkest through the fire, thou shalt not be burned, neither shall the flame kindle upon thee.

Ezekiel 33:3-4
3 if, when he seeth the sword come upon the land, he blow the trumpet, and warn the people;
4 then whosoever heareth the sound of the trumpet, and taketh not warning, if the sword come, and take him away, his blood shall be upon his own head.

Ezekiel 33:30-33
30 And as for thee, son of man, the children of thy people talk of thee by the walls and in the doors of the houses, and speak one to another, every one to his brother, saying, Come, I pray you, and hear what is the word that cometh forth from Jehovah.
31 And they come unto thee as the people cometh, and they sit before thee as my people, and they hear thy words, but do them not; for with their mouth they show much love, but their heart goeth after their gain.
32 And, lo, thou art unto them as a very lovely song of one that hath a pleasant voice, and can play well on an instrument; for they hear thy words, but they do them not.

33 And when this cometh to pass, (behold, it cometh,) then shall they know that a prophet hath been among them.

Zechariah 7:13
13 And it is come to pass that, as he cried, and they would not hear, so they shall cry, and I will not hear, said Jehovah of hosts;

Matthew 7:22-23
22 Many will say to me in that day, Lord, Lord, did we not prophesy by thy name, and by thy name cast out demons, and by thy name do many mighty works?
23 And then will I profess unto them, I never knew you: depart from me, ye that work iniquity.

Matthew 10:8
8 Heal the sick, raise the dead, cleanse the lepers, cast out demons: freely ye received, freely give.

Matthew 10:37
37 He that loveth father or mother more than me is not worthy of me; and he that loveth son or daughter more than me is not worthy of me.

Matthew 23:1-3
1 Then spake Jesus to the multitudes and to his disciples,
2 saying, The scribes and the Pharisees sit on Moses seat:
3 all things therefore whatsoever they bid you, these do and observe: but do not ye after their works; for they say, and do not.

Matthew 28:18
18 And Jesus came to them and spake unto them, saying, All authority hath been given unto me in heaven and on earth.

Luke 10:19
19 Behold, I have given you authority to tread upon serpents and scorpions, and over all the power of the enemy: and nothing shall in

any wise hurt you.

Luke 14:15
15 And when one of them that sat at meat with him heard these things, he said unto him, Blessed is he that shall eat bread in the kingdom of God.

John 3:36
36 He that believeth on the Son hath eternal life; but he that obeyeth not the Son shall not see life, but the wrath of God abideth on him.

John 7:17
17 If any man willeth to do his will, he shall know of the teaching, whether it is of God, or whether I speak from myself.

John 8:31-34
31 Jesus therefore said to those Jews that had believed him, If ye abide in my word, then are ye truly my disciples;
32 and ye shall know the truth, and the truth shall make you free.
33 They answered unto him, We are Abraham's seed, and have never yet been in bondage to any man: how sayest thou, Ye shall be made free?
34 Jesus answered them, Verily, verily, I say unto you, Every one that committeth sin is the bondservant of sin.

John 13:20
20 Verily, verily, I say unto you, he that receiveth whomsoever I send receiveth me; and he that receiveth me receiveth him that sent me.

John 15:6-10
6 If a man abide not in me, he is cast forth as a branch, and is withered; and they gather them, and cast them into the fire, and they are burned.
7 If ye abide in me, and my words abide in you, ask whatsoever ye will, and it shall be done unto you.
8 Herein is my Father glorified, that ye bear much fruit; and so shall

ye be my disciples.
9 Even as the Father hath loved me, I also have loved you: abide ye in my love.
10 If ye keep my commandments, ye shall abide in my love; even as I have kept my Father's commandments, and abide in his love.

Acts 23:5
5 And Paul said, I knew not, brethren, that he was high priest: for it is written, Thou shalt not speak evil of a ruler of thy people.

Romans 5:12
12 Therefore, as through one man sin entered into the world, and death through sin; and so death passed unto all men, for that all sinned.

Romans 6:16
16 Know ye not, that to whom ye present yourselves as servants unto obedience, his servants ye are whom ye obey; whether of sin unto death, or of obedience unto righteousness?

Romans 8:7
7 because the mind of the flesh is enmity against God; for it is not subject to the law of God, neither indeed can it be:

Romans 8:13
13 for if ye live after the flesh, ye must die; but if by the Spirit ye put to death the deeds of the body, ye shall live.

Romans 12:3-4
3 For I say, through the grace that was given me, to every man that is among you, not to think of himself more highly than he ought to think; but to think as to think soberly, according as God hath dealt to each man a measure of faith.
4 For even as we have many members in one body, and all the members have not the same office:

Romans 13:1-2

1 Let every soul be in subjection to the higher powers: for there is no power but of God; and the powers that be are ordained of God.
2 Therefore he that resisteth the power, withstandeth the ordinance of God: and they that withstand shall receive to themselves judgment.

Ephesians 5:23-24

23 For the husband is the head of the wife, and Christ also is the head of the church, being himself the saviour of the body.
24 But as the church is subject to Christ, so let the wives also be to their husbands in everything.

Colossians 3:20-25

20 Children, obey your parents in all things, for this is well-pleasing in the Lord.
21 Fathers, provoke not your children, that they be not discouraged.
22 Servants, obey in all things them that are your masters according to the flesh; not with eye-service, as men-pleasers, but in singleness of heart, fearing the Lord:
23 whatsoever ye do, work heartily, as unto the Lord, and not unto men;
24 knowing that from the Lord ye shall receive the recompense of the inheritance: ye serve the Lord Christ.
25 For he that doeth wrong shall receive again for the wrong that he hath done: and there is no respect of persons.

2 Thessalonians 2:10

10 and with all deceit of unrighteousness for them that perish; because they received not the love of the truth, that they might be saved.

1 Timothy 2:1-3

1 I exhort therefore, first of all, that supplications, prayers, intercessions, thanksgivings, be made for all men;
2 for kings and all that are in high place; that we may lead a tranquil

and quiet life in all godliness and gravity.
3 This is good and acceptable in the sight of God our Saviour;

1 Timothy 5:17
17 Let the elders that rule well be counted worthy of double honor, especially those who labor in the word and in teaching.

Titus 2:9-10
9 Exhort servants to be in subjection to their own masters, and to be well-pleasing to them in all things; not gainsaying;
10 not purloining, but showing all good fidelity; that they may adorn the doctrine of God our Saviour in all things.

Hebrews 11:6
6 And without faith it is impossible to be well-pleasing unto him; for he that cometh to God must believe that he is, and that he is a rewarder of them that seek after him.

Hebrews 12:1-3
1 Therefore let us also, seeing we are compassed about with so great a cloud of witnesses, lay aside every weight, and the sin which doth so easily beset us, and let us run with patience the race that is set before us,
2 looking unto Jesus the author and perfecter of our faith, who for the joy that was set before him endured the cross, despising shame, and hath sat down at the right hand of the throne of God.
3 For consider him that hath endured such gainsaying of sinners against himself, that ye wax not weary, fainting in your souls.

Hebrews 12:28
28 Wherefore, receiving a kingdom that cannot be shaken, let us have grace, whereby we may offer service well-pleasing to God with reverence and awe:

James 1:25
25 But he that looketh into the perfect law, the law of liberty, and

so continueth, being not a hearer that forgetteth but a doer that worketh, this man shall be blessed in his doing.

James 4:10
10 Humble yourselves in the sight of the Lord, and he shall exalt you.

1 Peter 1:17
17 And if ye call on him as Father, who without respect of persons judgeth according to each man's work, pass the time of your sojourning in fear:

1 Peter 2:11-13
11 Beloved, I beseech you as sojourners and pilgrims, to abstain from fleshly lust, which war against the soul;
12 having your behavior seemly among the Gentiles; that, wherein they speak against you as evil-doers, they may by your good works, which they behold, glorify God in the day of visitation.
13 Be subject to every ordinance of man for the Lord's sake: whether to the king, as supreme;

1 Peter 2:17-19
17 Honor all men. Love the brotherhood. Fear God. Honor the king.
18 Servants, be in subjection to your masters with all fear; not only to the good and gentle, but also to the froward.
19 For this is acceptable, if for conscience toward God a man endureth griefs, suffering wrongfully.

1 Peter 3:1
1 In like manner, ye wives, be in subjection to your won husbands; that, even if any obey not the word, they may without the word be gained by the behavior of their wives;

2 Peter 2:10
10 but chiefly them that walk after the flesh in the lust of defilement,

and despise dominion. Daring, self-willed, they tremble not to rail at dignities:

1 John 2:3-6

3 And hereby we know that we know him, if we keep his commandments.
4 He that saith, I know him, and keepeth not his commandments, is a liar, and the truth is not in him;
5 but whoso keepeth his word, in him verily hath the love of God been perfected. Hereby we know that we are in him:
6 he that saith he abideth in him ought himself also to walk even as he walked.

1 John 2:26-27

26 These things have I written unto you concerning them that would lead you astray.
27 And as for you, the anointing which ye received of him abideth in you, and ye need not that any one teach you; but as his anointing teacheth you; concerning all things, and is true, and is no lie, and even as it taught you, ye abide in him.

1 John 3:4

4 Every one that doeth sin doeth also lawlessness; and sin is lawlessness.

Our Helper: God's Spirit

It is God's intention to work through people. God gives each of us special gifts, which we are to develop with His help through experience and study. Unfortunately, compared to God, we are limited in knowledge and skills. So our prayers can open us up to allow God to accomplish those things in His will on our behalf. Sometimes all we have to do is ask! There are also times when we need assistance in an area of weakness. God knows this and wants to help us in those special times. You may need guidance with finding the right words in a delicate situation, or knowing what to do. Our daily lives are filled with hundreds of circumstances where we could use some direction or some answers.

The Holy Spirit is personal, for you and anyone else who will let Him operate in their life. Many fear God's Spirit, have little faith that the Holy Spirit can help, or have trouble being obedient to the Spirit. These are just some of the barriers you may be facing. If this is the case, you may need to visit a number of topics in this book in order to move forward. Moving forward in spiritual ways and receiving

God's blessing comes through exercising faith in Him. Yet this simple formula will be unique in how it works in your own life because we each come to God with a unique set of baggage—with differences in our life story, parental lines, knowledge base, and experiences. Our life can be changed for eternity only as we yield to God's written and living Word as it intercedes in and intercepts the course of our life.

> *Our life can be changed for eternity only as we yield to God's written and living Word as it intercedes in and intercepts the course of our life.*

Let me suggest that God's living Word be your guide as you use this book, whether you are praying for yourself or for others. Just ask God's Spirit for assistance. If you don't have a topic in mind, go to the index and scan the list until you feel drawn to one. Then go to that topic, scan the scripture, and pray with the verses you are drawn to. You may find that you are drawn to other topics as you proceed. This is good practice in seeing how the Holy Spirit wants to lead you through your daily life.

The Holy Spirit can assist you with the following:

- Directing you in prayer
- Teaching you His will for you
- Convicting you of sin in your life – OUCH!
- Helping you forgive someone who hurt you
- Putting boldness in your life
- Cutting through the fog of confusion
- Adding the fruits of the Spirit to your life: love, joy, peace, patience, kindness, goodness, faithfulness, gentleness, and self-control
- Understanding scripture
- Empowering you to live for Christ

Remember!
When praying scripture, give Jesus permission to search for lies and unbelief and replace them with God's truth.

Romans 13:2   Key Verse
2 Therefore he that resisteth the power, withstandeth the ordinance of God: and they that withstand shall receive to themselves judgment.

Psalms 143:10   Key Verse
10 Teach me to do thy will; For thou art my God: Thy Spirit is good; Lead me in the land of uprightness.

Romans 8:26-27   Key Verse
26 And in like manner the Spirit also helpeth our infirmity: for we know not how to pray as we ought; but the Spirit himself maketh intercession for us with groanings which cannot be uttered;
27 and he that searcheth the hearts knoweth what is the mind of the Spirit, because he maketh intercession for the saints according to the will of God.

Ephesians 3:20   Key Verse
20 Now unto him that is able to do exceeding abundantly above all that we ask or think, according to the power that worketh in us,

Psalms 10:14
14 Thou hast seen it; for thou beholdest mischief and spite, to requite it with thy hand: The helpless committeth himself unto thee; Thou hast been the helper of the fatherless.

Psalms 30:10
10 Hear, O Jehovah, and have mercy upon me: Jehovah, be thou my helper.

Psalms 54:4

4 Behold, God is my helper: The Lord is of them that uphold my soul.

Psalms 118:7

7 Jehovah is on my side among them that help me: Therefore shall I see my desire upon them that hate me.

Isaiah 28:11

11 Nay, but by men of strange lips and with another tongue will he speak to this people;

Isaiah 40:29

29 He giveth power to the faint; and to him that hath no might he increaseth strength.

Joel 2:28-29

28 And it shall come to pass afterward, that I will pour out my Spirit upon all flesh; and your sons and your daughters shall prophesy, your old men shall dream dreams, your young men shall see visions: 29 and also upon the servants and upon the handmaids in those days will I pour out my Spirit.

Matthew 3:11

11 I indeed baptize you in water unto repentance: but he that cometh after me is mightier than I, whose shoes I am not worthy to bear: he shall baptize you in the Holy Spirit and in fire:

Matthew 6:6

6 But thou, when thou prayest, enter into thine inner chamber, and having shut thy door, pray to thy Father who is in secret, and thy Father who seeth in secret shall recompense thee.

Matthew 9:8

8 But when the multitudes saw it, they were afraid, and glorified God, who had given such authority unto men.

Matthew 28:18

18 And Jesus came to them and spake unto them, saying, All authority hath been given unto me in heaven and on earth.

Mark 16:17

17 And these signs shall accompany them that believe: in my name shall they cast out demons; they shall speak with new tongues;

Acts 1:8

8 But ye shall receive power, when the Holy Spirit is come upon you: and ye shall be my witnesses both in Jerusalem, and in all Judaea and Samaria, and unto the uttermost part of the earth.

Luke 10:19

19 Behold, I have given you authority to tread upon serpents and scorpions, and over all the power of the enemy: and nothing shall in any wise hurt you.

Luke 11:13

13 If ye then, being evil, know how to give good gifts unto your children, how much more shall your heavenly Father give the Holy Spirit to them that ask him?

John 4:24

24 God is a Spirit: and they that worship him must worship in spirit and truth.

John 16:13-15

13 Howbeit when he, the Spirit of truth, is come, he shall guide you into all the truth: for he shall not speak from himself; but what things soever he shall hear, these shall he speak: and he shall declare unto you the things that are to come.
14 He shall glorify me: for he shall take of mine, and shall declare it unto you.
15 All things whatsoever the Father hath are mine: therefore said I, that he taketh of mine, and shall declare it unto you.

Acts 2:4

4 And they were all filled with the Holy Spirit, and began to speak with other tongues, as the Spirit gave them utterance.

Acts 10:45-46

45 And they of the circumcision that believed were amazed, as many as came with Peter, because that on the Gentiles also was poured out the gift of the Holy Spirit.
46 For they heard them speak with tongues, and magnify God. Then answered Peter,

Acts 2:16-17

16 but this is that which hath been spoken through the prophet Joel:
17 And it shall be in the last days, saith God, I will pour forth of My Spirit upon all flesh: And your sons and your daughters shall prophesy, And your young men shall see visions, And your old men shall dream

Acts 4:13

13 Now when they beheld the boldness of Peter and John, and had perceived that they were unlearned and ignorant men, they marvelled; and they took knowledge of them, that they had been with Jesus.
dreams:

Acts 4:29

29 And now, Lord, look upon their threatenings: and grant unto thy servants to speak thy word with all boldness,

Acts 8:19

19 saying, Give me also this power, that on whomsoever I lay my hands, he may receive the Holy Spirit.

Acts 19:2

2 and he said unto them, Did ye receive the Holy Spirit when ye believed? And they said unto him, Nay, we did not so much as hear whether the Holy Spirit was given.

Acts 19:6
6 And when Paul had laid his hands upon them, the Holy Spirit came on them; and they spake with tongues, and prophesied.

Romans 8:6
6 For the mind of the flesh is death; but the mind of the Spirit is life and peace:

Romans 8:13
13 for if ye live after the flesh, ye must die; but if by the Spirit ye put to death the deeds of the body, ye shall live.

Romans 15:13
13 Now the God of hope fill you with all joy and peace in believing, that ye may abound in hope, in the power of the Holy Spirit.

Romans 16:25
25 Now to him that is able to establish you according to my gospel and the preaching of Jesus Christ, according to the revelation of the mystery which hath been kept in silence through times eternal,

1 Corinthians 14:1-4
1 Follow after love; yet desire earnestly spiritual gifts, but rather that ye may prophesy.
2 For he that speaketh in a tongue speaketh not unto men, but unto God; for no man understandeth; but in the spirit he speaketh mysteries.
3 But he that prophesieth speaketh unto men edification, and exhortation, and consolation.
4 He that speaketh in a tongue edifieth himself; but he that prophesieth edifieth the church.

1 Corinthians 14:12-15

12 So also ye, since ye are zealous of spiritual gifts, seek that ye may abound unto the edifying of the church.
13 Wherefore let him that speaketh in a tongue pray that he may interpret.
14 For if I pray in a tongue, my spirit prayeth, but my understanding is unfruitful.
15 What is it then? I will pray with the spirit, and I will pray with the understanding also: I will sing with the spirit, and I will sing with the understanding also.

1 Corinthians 14:21

21 In the law it is written, By men of strange tongues and by the lips of strangers will I speak unto this people; and not even thus will they hear me, saith the Lord.

Galatians 5:22-23

22 But the fruit of the Spirit is love, joy, peace, longsuffering, kindness, goodness, faithfulness,
23 meekness, self-control; against such there is no law.

Philippians 1:20

20 according to my earnest expectation and hope, that in nothing shall I be put to shame, but that with all boldness, as always, so now also Christ shall be magnified in my body, whether by life, or by death.

1 Thessalonians 1:5

5 how that our gospel came not unto you in word only, but also in power, and in the Holy Spirit, and in much assurance; even as ye know what manner of men we showed ourselves toward you for your sake.

Ephesians 1:19

19 and what the exceeding greatness of his power to us-ward who believe, according to that working of the strength of his might

Ephesians 6:8
8 knowing that whatsoever good thing each one doeth, the same shall he receive again from the Lord, whether he be bond or free.

Ephesians 6:10
10 Finally, be strong in the Lord, and in the strength of his might.

Ephesians 6:18
18 with all prayer and supplication praying at all seasons in the Spirit, and watching thereunto in all perseverance and supplication for all the saints,

Hebrews 13:6
6 So that with good courage we say, The Lord is my helper; I will not fear: What shall man do unto me?

Hebrews 10:19
19 Having therefore, brethren, boldness to enter into the holy place by the blood of Jesus,

1 John 4:17
17 Herein is love made perfect with us, that we may have boldness in the day of judgment; because as he is, even so are we in this world.

Jude 1:20
20 But ye, beloved, building up yourselves on your most holy faith, praying in the Holy Spirit,

Overcoming Evil

It is said that the devil is defeated by the cross of Christ. When we think of the devil as being defeated, we think of the enemy as having lost its power. Yet he seems to be the instigator of so many problems during these last days. This is a difficult paradox.

Thus, I have come to understand that the devil gets his power from us. The Bible—God's Word—tells us to trust God. When we don't, we give the devil a way to control (power) us. Add unforgiveness, hate, guilt, shame and any other sin to our lack of faith, and this accounts for the open door we have given the devil to wreck havoc in our lives.

Unfortunately, the world has yielded a great amount of power to the devil, so in our intercessory responses for lost souls, we are still battling him. Jesus used scripture when in the desert, so we must conclude God's Word is our most effective weapon. I believe we must still pray in this manner because this is what we are shown in the New Testament, Ephesians 6:10-18, and in other verses.

It is also imperative that we maintain a personal faith connection to Christ. In Acts 19, certain vagabond Jews and seven sons of Sceva, who were a Jew and chief priest, tried to cast out a demon. But without their own personal relationship with Christ they were unable, and in fact, were injured in the process.

When praying during spiritual warfare, I believe we should keep in mind we are not really battling dark, evil spirits, but rather the grip they have individually or corporately. We are battling the mind, which is yielding to the world rather than to God. We are asking the Holy Spirit to soften hearts, to block negativity long enough so truth has an opportunity to shine its light in one's soul and spirit.

> *We are battling the mind, which is yielding to the world, rather than to God.*

Remember!
When praying scripture, give Jesus permission to search for lies and unbelief and replace them with God's truth.

Luke 10:19 Key Verse
19 Behold, I have given you authority to tread upon serpents and scorpions, and over all the power of the enemy: and nothing shall in any wise hurt you.

Ephesians 4:27 Key Verse
27 neither give place to the devil.

Romans 6:14 Key Verse
14 For sin shall not have dominion over you: for ye are not under law, but under grace.

1 John 4:6 (Falsehood / Error)   **Key Verse**
6 We are of God: he that knoweth God heareth us; he who is not of God heareth us not. By this we know the spirit of truth, and the spirit of error.

Genesis 6:4 (Sexual Activity)
4 The Nephilim were in the earth in those days, and also after that, when the sons of God came unto the daughters of men, and they bare children to them: the same were the mighty men that were of old, the men of renown.

Leviticus 26:40
40 And they shall confess their iniquity, and the iniquity of their fathers, in their trespass which they trespassed against me, and also that, because they walked contrary unto me,

Leviticus 26:42
42 then will I remember my covenant with Jacob; and also my covenant with Isaac, and also my covenant with Abraham will I remember; and I will remember the land.

Numbers 5:14 (Jealousy)
14 and the spirit of jealousy come upon him, and he be jealous of his wife, and she be defiled: or if the spirit of jealousy come upon him, and he be jealous of his wife, and she be not defiled:

Numbers 5:30 (Jealousy)
30 or when the spirit of jealousy cometh upon a man, and he is jealous of his wife; then shall he set the woman before Jehovah, and the priest shall execute upon her all this law.

Deuteronomy 18:11 (Familiar Spirits)
11 or a charmer, or a consulter with a familiar spirit, or a wizard, or a necromancer.

Deuteronomy 32:20
20 And he said, I will hide my face from them, I will see what their end shall be: For they are a very perverse generation, Children in whom is no faithfulness.

Judges 9:23 (Treachery)
23 And God sent an evil spirit between Abimelech and the men of Shechem; and the men of Shechem dealt treacherously with Abimelech:

1 Samuel 1:10 (Sorrow or Bitterness)
10 And she was in bitterness of soul, and prayed unto Jehovah, and wept sore.

1 Samuel 13:8-14
8 And he tarried seven days, according to the set time that Samuel had appointed: but Samuel came not to Gilgal; and the people were scattered from him.
9 And Saul said, Bring hither the burnt-offering to me, and the peace-offerings. And he offered the burnt-offering.
10 And it came to pass that, as soon as he had made an end of offering the burnt-offering, behold, Samuel came; and Saul went out to meet him, that he might salute him.
11 And Samuel said, What hast thou done? And Saul said, Because I saw that the people were scattered from me, and that thou camest not within the days appointed, and that the Philistines assembled themselves together at Michmash;
12 therefore said I, Now will the Philistines come down upon me to Gilgal, and I have not entreated the favor of Jehovah: I forced myself therefore, and offered the burnt-offering.
13 And Samuel said to Saul, Thou hast done foolishly; thou hast not kept the commandment of Jehovah thy God, which he commanded thee: for now would Jehovah have established thy kingdom upon Israel for ever.
14 But now thy kingdom shall not continue: Jehovah hath sought him a man after his own heart, and Jehovah hath appointed him

to be prince over his people, because thou hast not kept that which Jehovah commanded thee.

1 Samuel 15:14-23 (Rebellion)
14 And Samuel said, What meaneth then this bleating of the sheep in mine ears, and the lowing of the oxen which I hear?
15 And Saul said, They have brought them from the Amalekites: for the people spared the best of the sheep and of the oxen, to sacrifice unto Jehovah thy God; and the rest we have utterly destroyed.
16 Then Samuel said unto Saul, Stay, and I will tell thee what Jehovah hath said to me this night. And he said unto him, Say on.
17 And Samuel said, Though thou wast little in thine own sight, wast thou not made the head of the tribes of Israel? And Jehovah anointed thee king over Israel;
18 and Jehovah sent thee on a journey, and said, Go, and utterly destroy the sinners the Amalekites, and fight against them until they be consumed.
19 Wherefore then didst thou not obey the voice of Jehovah, but didst fly upon the spoil, and didst that which was evil in the sight of Jehovah?
20 And Saul said unto Samuel, Yea, I have obeyed the voice of Jehovah, and have gone the way which Jehovah sent me, and have brought Agag the king of Amalek, and have utterly destroyed the Amalekites.
21 But the people took of the spoil, sheep and oxen, the chief of the devoted things, to sacrifice unto Jehovah thy God in Gilgal.
22 And Samuel said, Hath Jehovah as great delight in burnt-offerings and sacrifices, as in obeying the voice of Jehovah? Behold, to obey is better than sacrifice, and to hearken than the fat of rams.
23 For rebellion is as the sin of witchcraft, and stubbornness is as idolatry and teraphim. Because thou hast rejected the word of Jehovah, he hath also rejected thee from being king.

1 Samuel 16:14 (Injurious Spirit)
14 Now the Spirit of Jehovah departed from Saul, and an evil spirit from Jehovah troubled him.

1 Samuel 28:3 (Familiar Spirits)
3 Now Samuel was dead, and all Israel had lamented him, and buried him in Ramah, even in his own city. And Saul had put away those that had familiar spirits, and the wizards, out of the land.

1 Kings 22:21-23 (Lying Spirit)
21 And there came forth a spirit, and stood before Jehovah, and said, I will entice him.
22 And Jehovah said unto him, Wherewith? And he said, I will go forth, and will be a lying spirit in the mouth of all his prophets. And he said, Thou shalt entice him, and shalt prevail also: go forth, and do so.
23 Now therefore, behold, Jehovah hath put a lying spirit in the mouth of all these thy prophets; and Jehovah hath spoken evil concerning thee.

2 Kings 23:24 (Familiar Spirits)
24 Moreover them that had familiar spirits, and the wizards, and the teraphim, and the idols, and all the abominations that were seen in the land of Judah and in Jerusalem, did Josiah put away, that he might confirm the words of the law which were written in the book that Hilkiah the priest found in the house of Jehovah.

2 Chronicles 7:14
14 if my people, who are called by my name, shall humble themselves, and pray, and seek my face, and turn from their wicked ways; then will I hear from heaven, and will forgive their sin, and will heal their land.

Psalms 91:11
11 For he will give his angels charge over thee, To keep thee in all thy ways.

Proverbs 16:18 (Pride)
18 Pride goeth before destruction, And a haughty spirit before a fall.

Proverbs 28:13
13 He that covereth his transgressions shall not prosper: But whoso confesseth and forsaketh them shall obtain mercy.

Isaiah 8:9 (ASV) (Familiar Spirits)
9 Make an uproar, O ye peoples, and be broken in pieces; and give ear, all ye of far countries: gird yourselves, and be broken in pieces; gird yourselves, and be broken in pieces.

Isaiah 19:14 (Confusion)
14 Jehovah hath mingled a spirit of perverseness in the midst of her; and they have caused Egypt to go astray in every work thereof, as a drunken man staggereth in his vomit.

Isaiah 29:10 (Slumber or Deep Sleep / Blindness to Truth)
10 For Jehovah hath poured out upon you the spirit of deep sleep, and hath closed your eyes, the prophets; and your heads, the seers, hath he covered.

Isaiah 47:1-3 (Jezebel)
1 Come down, and sit in the dust, O virgin daughter of Babylon; sit on the ground without a throne, O daughter of the Chaldeans: for thou shalt no more be called tender and delicate.
2 Take the millstones, and grind meal; remove thy veil, strip off the train, uncover the leg, pass through the rivers.
3 Thy nakedness shall be uncovered, yea, thy shame shall be seen: I will take vengeance, and will spare no man.

Isaiah 54:17
17 No weapon that is formed against thee shall prosper; and every tongue that shall rise against thee in judgment thou shalt condemn. This is the heritage of the servants of Jehovah, and their righteousness which is of me, saith Jehovah.

Isaiah 61:3 (Heaviness / Despair)
3 to appoint unto them that mourn in Zion, to give unto them

a garland for ashes, the oil of joy for mourning, the garment of praise for the spirit of heaviness; that they may be called trees of righteousness, the planting of Jehovah, that he may be glorified.

Zechariah 13:2 (Spirit of Impurity)
2 And it shall come to pass in that day, saith Jehovah of hosts, that I will cut off the names of the idols out of the land, and they shall no more be remembered; and also I will cause the prophets and the unclean spirit to pass out of the land.

Matthew 8:16-17 (Infirmities)
16 And when even was come, they brought unto him many possessed with demons: and he cast out the spirits with a word, and healed all that were sick:
17 that it might be fulfilled which was spoken through Isaiah the prophet, saying: Himself took our infirmities, and bare our diseases.

Matthew 9:32-33 (Dumb Spirit)
32 And as they went forth, behold, there was brought to him a dumb man possessed with a demon.
33 And when the demon was cast out, the dumb man spake: and the multitudes marvelled, saying, It was never so seen in Israel.

Matthew 12:29
29 Or how can one enter into the house of the strong man, and spoil his goods, except he first bind the strong man? and then he will spoil his house.

Matthew 18:18
18 Verily I say unto you, what things soever ye shall bind on earth shall be bound in heaven; and what things soever ye shall loose on earth shall be loosed in heaven.

Matthew 22:29
29 But Jesus answered and said unto them, Ye do err, not knowing

the scriptures, nor the power of God.

Mark 7:25 (Unclean / Impure)
25 But straightway a woman, whose little daughter had an unclean spirit, having heard of him, came and fell down at his feet.

Mark 9:22 (Injury and Death)
22 And oft-times it hath cast him both into the fire and into the waters, to destroy him: but if thou canst do anything, have compassion on us, and help us.

Mark 9:25 (Dumb Spirit)
25 And when Jesus saw that a multitude came running together, he rebuked the unclean spirit, saying unto him, Thou dumb and deaf spirit, I command thee, come out of him, and enter no more into him.

Luke 5:15 (Sickness)
15 But so much the more went abroad the report concerning him: and great multitudes came together to hear, and to be healed of their infirmities.

Luke 7:21 (Evil Spirits)
21 In that hour he cured many of diseases and plagues and evil spirits; and on many that were blind he bestowed sight.

Luke 8:2 (Disease)
2 and certain women who had been healed of evil spirits and infirmities: Mary that was called Magdalene, from whom seven demons had gone out,

Luke 8:26-39 (Insanity / Decency / Violence)
26 And they arrived at the country of the Gerasenes, which is over against Galilee.
27 And when he was come forth upon the land, there met him a certain man out of the city, who had demons; and for a long time

he had worn no clothes, and abode not in any house, but in the tombs.

28 And when he saw Jesus, he cried out, and fell down before him, and with a loud voice said, What have I to do with thee, Jesus, thou Son of the Most High God? I beseech thee, torment me not.

29 For he was commanding the unclean spirit to come out from the man. For oftentimes it had seized him: and he was kept under guard, and bound with chains and fetters; and breaking the bands asunder, he was driven of the demon into the deserts.

30 And Jesus asked him, What is thy name? And he said, Legion; for many demons were entered into him.

31 And they entreated him that he would not command them to depart into the abyss.

32 Now there was a herd of many swine feeding on the mountain: and they entreated him that he would give them leave to enter into them. And he gave them leave.

33 And the demons came out from the man, and entered into the swine: and the herd rushed down the steep into the lake, and were drowned.

34 And when they that fed them saw what had come to pass, they fled, and told it in the city and in the country.

35 And they went out to see what had come to pass; and they came to Jesus, and found the man, from whom the demons were gone out, sitting, clothed and in his right mind, at the feet of Jesus: and they were afraid.

36 And they that saw it told them how he that was possessed with demons was made whole.

37 And all the people of the country of the Gerasenes round about asked him to depart from them, for they were holden with great fear: and he entered into a boat, and returned.

38 But the man from whom the demons were gone out prayed him that he might be with him: but he sent him away, saying,

39 Return to thy house, and declare how great things God hath done for thee. And he went his way, publishing throughout the whole city how great things Jesus had done for him.

Luke 13:11 (Crippling Spirit)
11 And behold, a woman that had a spirit of infirmity eighteen years; and she was bowed together, and could in no wise lift herself up.

Luke 11:4
4 And forgive us our sins; for we ourselves also forgive every one that is indebted to us. And bring us not into temptation.

John 5:5 (Invalidity)
5 And a certain man was there, who had been thirty and eight years in his infirmity.

John 17:15
15 I pray not that thou shouldest take them from the world, but that thou shouldest keep them from the evil one.

Acts 16:16 (Divination)
16 And it came to pass, as we were going to the place of prayer, that a certain maid having a spirit of divination met us, who brought her masters much gain by soothsaying.

Acts 19:12 (Evil Spirits)
12 insomuch that unto the sick were carried away from his body handkerchiefs or aprons, and the evil spirits went out.

Romans 6:6
6 knowing this, that our old man was crucified with him, that the body of sin might be done away, that so we should no longer be in bondage to sin;

Romans 6:11
11 Even so reckon ye also yourselves to be dead unto sin, but alive unto God in Christ Jesus.

Romans 8:37

37 Nay, in all these things we are more than conquerors through him that loved us.

Romans 11:26

26 and so all Israel shall be saved: even as it is written, There shall come out of Zion the Deliverer; He shall turn away ungodliness from Jacob:

1 Corinthians 1:27

27 but God chose the foolish things of the world, that he might put to shame them that are wise; and God chose the weak things of the world, that he might put to shame the things that are strong;

Galatians 3:13-14

13 Christ redeemed us from the curse of the law, having become a curse for us; for it is written, Cursed is every one that hangeth on a tree:
14 that upon the Gentiles might come the blessing of Abraham in Christ Jesus; that we might receive the promise of the Spirit through faith.

Ephesians 1:19-21

19 and what the exceeding greatness of his power to us-ward who believe, according to that working of the strength of his might
20 which he wrought in Christ, when he raised him from the dead, and made him to sit at his right hand in the heavenly places,
21 far above all rule, and authority, and power, and dominion, and every name that is named, not only in this world, but also in that which is to come:

Ephesians 6:10-12

10 Finally, be strong in the Lord, and in the strength of his might.
11 Put on the whole armor of God, that ye may be able to stand against the wiles of the devil.
12 For our wrestling is not against flesh and blood, but against the

principalities, against the powers, against the world-rulers of this darkness, against the spiritual hosts of wickedness in the heavenly places.

Colossians 1:13-14
13 who delivered us out of the power of darkness, and translated us into the kingdom of the Son of his love;
14 in whom we have our redemption, the forgiveness of our sins:

Colossians 2:13-14
13 And you, being dead through your trespasses and the uncircumcision of your flesh, you, I say, did he make alive together with him, having forgiven us all our trespasses;
14 having blotted out the bond written in ordinances that was against us, which was contrary to us: and he hath taken it out that way, nailing it to the cross;

Colossians 2:9-10 (Head of Power)
9 for in him dwelleth all the fulness of the Godhead bodily,
10 and in him ye are made full, who is the head of all principality and power:

Colossians 3:3 (Hidden from Satan)
3 For ye died, and your life is hid with Christ in God.

1 Timothy 4:1 (Unbelief)
1 But the Spirit saith expressly, that in later times some shall fall away from the faith, giving heed to seducing spirits and doctrines of demons,

Titus 2:14
14 who gave himself for us, that he might redeem us from all iniquity, and purify unto himself a people for his own possession, zealous of good works.

Hebrews 2:14

14 Since then the children are sharers in flesh and blood, he also himself in like manner partook of the same; that through death he might bring to nought him that had the power of death, that is, the devil;

James 4:6-7

6 But he giveth more grace. Wherefore the scripture saith, God resisteth the proud, but giveth grace to the humble.
7 Be subject therefore unto God; but resist the devil, and he will flee from you.

1 John 4:1-3 (Antichrist)

1 Beloved, believe not every spirit, but prove the spirits, whether they are of God; because many false prophets are gone out into the world.
2 Hereby know ye the Spirit of God: every spirit that confesseth that Jesus Christ is come in the flesh is of God:
3 and every spirit that confesseth not Jesus is not of God: and this is the spirit of the antichrist, whereof ye have heard that it cometh; and now it is in the world already.

1 John 4:9

9 Herein was the love of God manifested in us, that God hath sent his only begotten Son into the world that we might live through him.

Revelation 17:4 (Unclean / Impure)

4 And the woman was arrayed in purple and scarlet, and decked with gold and precious stone and pearls, having in her hand a golden cup full of abominations, even the unclean things of her fornication,

Peace and Stress

Jesus is called the Prince of Peace. Nowhere is that more evident than the time Jesus and His disciples were in a boat crossing the lake when a fierce storm arose. Fearfully, the disciples woke Jesus, who rebuked the wind and waves. Suddenly, there was great calm. Just as Jesus calmed the storm on the lake, He can calm the storms in your life.

> *Jesus will bring peace to our life, but remember that peace comes after facing the storm.*

Many situations can stir us up and create all kinds of stress. Childhood wounds and trauma may be relived as daily events trigger memories of the past. While we may not consciously remember the actual events, they are recorded someplace in our memory.

Mindsets of fear, hate, etc., linger in our life, keeping us out of ease. Jesus will bring peace to our life, but remember that peace comes after facing the storm. You need to be attentive to where Jesus wants to send you. This inner turmoil can have multiple sources, so as we deal with various issues, our life becomes more peaceful. We might say that when we don't have ease in our life, our life is at dis-ease!

Stress
Stressors are those things that put adverse pressure on our lives. Although a stressor can be something physical, such as an extreme temperature, for the purpose of this discussion we are primarily concerned with mental stress. Our job, finances, and family situations can all be stressful. There is even a test that rates stress factors such as losing a job, moving, a death in the family, divorce, and more. We all handle stress differently, however, those who can turn their daily worries over to God fare much better.

There is another aspect of stress not connected to our present life and current events, and that is the stress of the past. Past events which caused us to feel fear can be a continuous source of anxiety. Lingering feelings of shame, guilt, hopelessness, unworthiness, and other lies of the enemy can steal our peace and become ongoing sources of stress.

Medical science has found that the emotional impact of childhood neglect, abuse, or trauma can not only be a source of stress in our life, but lead to morbidity, mortality, and obesity. Simply put, stress is a peace destroyer. Start to bring more peace into your life today by praying with the appropriate scripture verses. Ask the Lord to replace the lies with His truth.

Remember!
When praying scripture, give Jesus permission to search for lies and unbelief and replace them with God's truth.

2 Thessalonians 3:16 Key Verse
16 Now the Lord of peace himself give you peace at all times in all ways. The Lord be with you all.

Psalms 138:7 Key Verse
7 Though I walk in the midst of trouble, thou wilt revive me; Thou wilt stretch forth thy hand against the wrath of mine enemies, And thy right hand will save me.

John 14:27 Key Verse
27 Peace I leave with you; my peace I give unto you: not as the world giveth, give I unto you. Let not your heart be troubled, neither let it be fearful.

Numbers 6:24-26
24 Jehovah bless thee, and keep thee:
25 Jehovah make his face to shine upon thee, and be gracious unto thee:
26 Jehovah lift up his countenance upon thee, and give thee peace.

Psalms 22:24
24 For he hath not despised nor abhorred the affliction of the afflicted; Neither hath he hid his face from him; But when he cried unto him, he heard.

Colossians 3:15
15 And let the peace of Christ rule in your hearts, to the which also ye were called in one body; and be ye thankful.

Psalms 27:14
14 Wait for Jehovah: Be strong, And let thy heart take courage; Yea, wait thou for Jehovah.

Psalms 29:11
11 Jehovah will give strength unto his people; Jehovah will bless his people with peace.

Psalms 46:10
10 Be still, and know that I am God: I will be exalted among the nations, I will be exalted in the earth.

Psalms 119:165

165 Great peace have they that love thy law; And they have no occasion of stumbling.

Proverbs 1:33

33 But whoso hearkeneth unto me shall dwell securely, And shall be quiet without fear of evil.

Isaiah 26:3

3 Thou wilt keep him in perfect peace, whose mind is stayed on thee; because he trusteth in thee.

Matthew 11:28-29

28 Come unto me, all ye that labor and are heavy laden, and I will give you rest.
29 Take my yoke upon you, and learn of me; for I am meek and lowly in heart: and ye shall find rest unto your souls.

Mark 4:39

39 And he awoke, and rebuked the wind, and said unto the sea, Peace, be still. And the wind ceased, and there was a great calm.

John 16:33

33 These things have I spoken unto you, that in me ye may have peace. In the world ye have tribulation: but be of good cheer; I have overcome the world.

Romans 5:1-2

1 Being therefore justified by faith, we have peace with God through our Lord Jesus Christ;
2 through whom also we have had our access by faith into this grace wherein we stand; and we rejoice in hope of the glory of God.

Philippians 4:6

6 In nothing be anxious; but in everything by prayer and supplication with thanksgiving let your requests be made known unto God.

2 John 1:3

3 Grace, mercy, peace shall be with us, from God the Father, and from Jesus Christ, the Son of the Father, in truth and love.

Prayer And Difficulty Praying

Our access to God's blessings and help is through prayer. There are many books that explain all aspects of prayer, and you can gain much insight and knowledge by reading them. If prayer is difficult for you, the power of God's Word may be very helpful. We all need to connect with God and be in His presence. You may find it beneficial to read and pray Psalm 91 in its entirety from your Bible, which is about being in God's presence. Another idea that may be helpful is going to the topic "overcoming evil" and pray scripture verses appropriate to your situation.

 Remember!
When praying scripture, give Jesus permission to search for lies and unbelief and replace them with God's truth.

Matthew 7:7   Key Verse
7 Ask, and it shall be given you; seek, and ye shall find; knock, and

it shall be opened unto you:

Matthew 26:41   Key Verse
41 Watch and pray, that ye enter not into temptation: the spirit indeed is willing, but the flesh is weak.

Luke 11:10   Key Verse
10 For every one that asketh receiveth; and he that seeketh findeth; and to him that knocketh it shall be opened.

Deuteronomy 4:29
29 But from thence ye shall seek Jehovah thy God, and thou shalt find him, when thou searchest after him with all thy heart and with all thy soul.

1 Chronicles 16:11
11 Seek ye Jehovah and his strength; Seek his face evermore.

2 Chronicles 7:14
14 if my people, who are called by my name, shall humble themselves, and pray, and seek my face, and turn from their wicked ways; then will I hear from heaven, and will forgive their sin, and will heal their land.

Psalms 65:2
2 O thou that hearest prayer, Unto thee shall all flesh come.

Psalms 145:18
18 Jehovah is nigh unto all them that call upon him, To all that call upon him in truth.

Proverbs 28:9
9 He that turneth away his ear from hearing the law, Even his prayer is an abomination.

Isaiah 56:7
7 even them will I bring to my holy mountain, and make them joyful in my house of prayer: their burnt-offerings and their sacrifices shall be accepted upon mine altar; for my house shall be called a house of prayer for all peoples.

Jeremiah 29:13
13 And ye shall seek me, and find me, when ye shall search for me with all your heart.

Ezekiel 36:37
37 Thus saith the Lord Jehovah: For this, moreover, will I be inquired of by the house of Israel, to do it for them: I will increase them with men like a flock.

Hosea 14:2
2 Take with you words, and return unto Jehovah: say unto him, Take away all iniquity, and accept that which is good: so will we render as bullocks the offering of our lips.

Micah 3:4
4 Then shall they cry unto Jehovah, but he will not answer them; yea, he will hide his face from them at that time, according as they have wrought evil in their doings.

Matthew 21:22
22 And all things, whatsoever ye shall ask in prayer, believing, ye shall receive.

Mark 9:23
23 And Jesus said unto him, If thou canst! All things are possible to him that believeth.

Mark 11:23-24
23 Verily I say unto you, Whosoever shall say unto this mountain, Be thou taken up and cast into the sea; and shall not doubt in his

heart, but shall believe that what he saith cometh to pass; he shall have it.

24 Therefore I say unto you, All things whatsoever ye pray and ask for, believe that ye receive them, and ye shall have them.

Luke 6:28
28 bless them that curse you, pray for them that despitefully use you.

Luke 11:12
12 Or if he shall ask an egg, will he give him a scorpion?

Luke 11:13
13 If ye then, being evil, know how to give good gifts unto your children, how much more shall your heavenly Father give the Holy Spirit to them that ask him?

Luke 22:40
40 And when he was at the place, he said unto them, Pray that ye enter not into temptation.

Romans 8:6
6 For the mind of the flesh is death; but the mind of the Spirit is life and peace:

Romans 12:12
12 rejoicing in hope; patient in tribulation; continuing stedfastly in prayer;

1 Corinthians 2:11-13
11 For who among men knoweth the things of a man, save the spirit of the man, which is in him? even so the things of God none knoweth, save the Spirit of God. 12 But we received, not the spirit of the world, but the spirit which is from God; that we might know the things that were freely given to us of God.

13 Which things also we speak, not in words which man's wisdom teacheth, but which the Spirit teacheth; combining spiritual things with spiritual words.

Colossians 4:2
2 Continue stedfastly in prayer, watching therein with thanksgiving;

James 1:6-7
6 But let him ask in faith, nothing doubting: for he that doubteth is like the surge of the sea driven by the wind and tossed.
7 For let not that man think that he shall receive anything of the Lord;

James 4:3
3 Ye ask, and receive not, because ye ask amiss, that ye may spend it in your pleasures.

James 5:13
13 Is any among you suffering? Let him pray. Is any cheerful? Let him sing praise.

James 5:16
16 Confess therefore your sins one to another, and pray one for another, that ye may be healed. The supplication of a righteous man availeth much in its working.

1 John 3:22
22 and whatsoever we ask we receive of him, because we keep his commandments and do the things that are pleasing in his sight.

1 John 5:14
14 And this is the boldness which we have toward him, that, if we ask anything according to his will, he heareth us:

Pride

Proverbs 16:18 reads: "*Pride goes before destruction, and a haughty spirit before a fall.*" With pride, we see a level of arrogance in which people project superiority over others. The humanist movement equates itself with God. Prideful people can be judgmental, while oblivious to their own shortcomings.

Judging people is one attribute of pride, and of course, God has something to say about judging.

Matthew 7:1-5
1 Judge not, that ye be not judged. 2 For with what judgment ye judge, ye shall be judged: and with what measure ye mete, it shall be measured unto you. 3 And why beholdest thou the mote that is in thy brother's eye, but considerest not the beam that is in thine own eye? 4 Or how wilt thou say to thy brother, Let me cast out the mote out of thine eye; and lo, the beam is in thine own eye? 5 Thou hypocrite, cast out first the beam out of thine own eye; and then shalt thou see clearly to cast out the mote out of thy brother's eye.

Pride allows us to justify sin or have our own pity party. It is a big obstacle in letting God into our life to help us along the path of transformation. Without transformation, our lives will stay fairly stagnant. And don't be envious of those whose lives are changing, as evidenced by the unmistakable outer joy they display.

> *Pride allows us to justify sin or have our own pity party.*

Some may say, "I'm not prideful; people tell me how they appreciate my humbleness." Be careful, you may be exhibiting a false humbleness that is covering up true feelings of pride. It could be the result of choices influenced by a very poor self-esteem, and a person who doesn't know their identity and value in Christ. God values all of us. Knowing this is foundational to liking ourselves. When we don't like ourselves, we tend to do things that are self-destructive. Sometimes it's an attitude of "I can do it myself." Isn't that what our culture encourages and the principle upon which our country was founded? Most likely, the attitude of self-sufficiency formed from watching our parents and others as we were growing up. Another possibility is that when we have been seriously hurt as children, anger begins to fester in us, leading to rebellion. For many of the founding fathers, their resolve was *because* of their faith and reliance upon God, not in spite of it.

People hurt as children usually are angry at their perpetrators, which is understandable. They also can become angry at God for not protecting them. Why didn't this all-powerful God intervene? The answer is God doesn't interfere with people even when they are doing evil. Not only does this reinforce the stronghold of anger, but also the stronghold of pride in self-suffering. In effect, the victim is telling the perpetrator, "You broke me, so fix me." When the anger is transferred to God, in essence, it is God who must fix us now. The truth is, nothing changes until we act by opening the door for God.

The point is that if you rely only on yourself, there will be no room in your life for God and His life-changing power. If you want to move forward, you may need to spend some time in prayer with the following scripture verses. Don't forget that Jesus sent the Holy Spirit to help us. Be bold—ask for help.

Remember!
When praying scripture, give Jesus permission to search for lies and unbelief and replace them with God's truth.

Proverbs 16:18-19   Key Verse
18 Pride goeth before destruction, And a haughty spirit before a fall.
19 Better it is to be of a lowly spirit with the poor, Than to divide the spoil with the proud.

Job 35:12   Key Verse
12 There they cry, but none giveth answer, Because of the pride of evil men.

James 4:6b   Key Verse
6b God resisteth the proud, but giveth grace to the humble.

1 Timothy 3:6   Key Verse
6 not a novice, lest being puffed up he fall into the condemnation of the devil.

Leviticus 26:19
19 And I will break the pride of your power: and I will make your heaven as iron, and your earth as brass;

Deuteronomy 8:18

18 But thou shalt remember Jehovah thy God, for it is he that giveth thee power to get wealth; that he may establish his covenant which he sware unto thy fathers, as at this day.

2 Chronicles 26:16-21

16 But when he was strong, his heart was lifted up, so that he did corruptly, and he trespassed against Jehovah his God; for he went into the temple of Jehovah to burn incense upon the altar of incense.

17 And Azariah the priest went in after him, and with him fourscore priests of Jehovah, that were valiant men: 18 and they withstood Uzziah the king, and said unto him, It pertaineth not unto thee, Uzziah, to burn incense unto Jehovah, but to the priests the sons of Aaron, that are consecrated to burn incense: go out of the sanctuary; for thou hast trespassed; neither shall it be for thine honor from Jehovah God.

19 Then Uzziah was wroth; and he had a censer in his hand to burn incense; and while he was wroth with the priests, the leprosy brake forth in his forehead before the priests in the house of Jehovah, beside the altar of incense. 20 And Azariah the chief priest, and all the priests, looked upon him, and, behold, he was leprous in his forehead, and they thrust him out quickly from thence; yea, himself hasted also to go out, because Jehovah had smitten him. 21 And Uzziah the king was a leper unto the day of his death, and dwelt in a separate house, being a leper; for he was cut off from the house of Jehovah: and Jotham his son was over the king's house, judging the people of the land.

Psalms 10:2

2 In the pride of the wicked the poor is hotly pursued; Let them be taken in the devices that they have conceived.

Psalms 10:4

4 The wicked, in the pride of his countenance, saith, He will not require it. All his thoughts are, There is no God

Psalms 36:11
11 Let not the foot of pride come against me, And let not the hand of the wicked drive me away.

Psalms 73:6
6 Therefore pride is as a chain about their neck; Violence covereth them as a garment.

Psalms 119:113
113 I hate them that are of a double mind; But thy law do I love.

Proverbs 8:13
13 The fear of Jehovah is to hate evil: Pride, and arrogancy, and the evil way, And the perverse mouth, do I hate.

Proverbs 11:2
2 When pride cometh, then cometh shame; But with the lowly is wisdom.

Proverbs 13:10
10 By pride cometh only contention; But with the well-advised is wisdom.

Proverbs 14:3
3 In the mouth of the foolish is a rod for his pride; But the lips of the wise shall preserve them.

Proverbs 23:7
7 For as he thinketh within himself, so is he: Eat and drink, saith he to thee; But his heart is not with thee.

Proverbs 29:23
23 A man's pride shall bring him low; But he that is of a lowly spirit shall obtain honor.

Isaiah 9:8-9

*8 The Lord sent a word into Jacob, and it hath lighted upon Israel.
9 And all the people shall know, even Ephraim and the inhabitant of Samaria, that say in pride and in stoutness of heart,*

Isaiah 14:12-15

*12 How art thou fallen from heaven, O day-star, son of the morning! how art thou cut down to the ground, that didst lay low the nations!
13 And thou saidst in thy heart, I will ascend into heaven, I will exalt my throne above the stars of God; and I will sit upon the mount of congregation, in the uttermost parts of the north;
14 I will ascend above the heights of the clouds; I will make myself like the Most High.
15 Yet thou shalt be brought down to Sheol, to the uttermost parts of the pit.*

Isaiah 16:6

6 We have heard of the pride of Moab, that he is very proud; even of his arrogancy, and his pride, and his wrath; his boastings are nought.

Isaiah 25:11

11 And he shall spread forth his hands in the midst thereof, as he that swimmeth spreadeth forth his hands to swim; but Jehovah will lay low his pride together with the craft of his hands.

Jeremiah 13:9

9 Thus saith Jehovah, After this manner will I mar the pride of Judah, and the great pride of Jerusalem.

Jeremiah 13:17

17 But if ye will not hear it, my soul shall weep in secret for your pride; and mine eye shall weep sore, and run down with tears, because Jehovah's flock is taken captive.

Jeremiah 49:16

16 As for thy terribleness, the pride of thy heart hath deceived thee, O thou that dwellest in the clefts of the rock, that holdest the height of the hill: though thou shouldest make thy nest as high as the eagle, I will bring thee down from thence, saith Jehovah.

Ezekiel 28:1-2

1 The word of Jehovah came again unto me, saying,
2 Son of man, say unto the prince of Tyre, Thus saith the Lord Jehovah: Because thy heart is lifted up, and thou hast said, I am a god, I sit in the seat of God, in the midst of the seas; yet thou art man, and not God, though thou didst set thy heart as the heart of God;--

Ezekiel 30:6

6 Thus saith Jehovah: They also that uphold Egypt shall fall; and the pride of her power shall come down: from the tower of Seveneh shall they fall in it by the sword, saith the Lord Jehovah.

Daniel 4:37

37 Now I, Nebuchadnezzar, praise and extol and honor the King of heaven; for all his works are truth, and his ways justice; and those that walk in pride he is able to abase.

Daniel 4:34-35

34 And at the end of the days I, Nebuchadnezzar, lifted up mine eyes unto heaven, and mine understanding returned unto me, and I blessed the Most High, and I praised and honored him that liveth for ever; for his dominion is an everlasting dominion, and his kingdom from generation to generation.
35 And all the inhabitants of the earth are reputed as nothing; and he doeth according to his will in the army of heaven, and among the inhabitants of the earth; and none can stay his hand, or say unto him, What doest thou?

Daniel 5:20

20 But when his heart was lifted up, and his spirit was hardened so that he dealt proudly, he was deposed from his kingly throne, and they took his glory from him:

Hosea 5:5

5 And the pride of Israel doth testify to his face: therefore Israel and Ephraim shall stumble in their iniquity; Judah also shall stumble with them.

Hosea 7:10

10 And the pride of Israel doth testify to his face: yet they have not returned unto Jehovah their God, nor sought him, for all this.

Luke 17:7-10

7 But who is there of you, having a servant plowing or keeping sheep, that will say unto him, when he is come in from the field, Come straightway and sit down to meat;
8 and will not rather say unto him, Make ready wherewith I may sup, and gird thyself, and serve me, till I have eaten and drunken; and afterward thou shalt eat and drink?
9 Doth he thank the servant because he did the things that were commanded?
10 Even so ye also, when ye shall have done all the things that are commanded you, say, We are unprofitable servants; we have done that which it was our duty to do.

Acts 12:20-23

20 Now he was highly displeased with them of Tyre and Sidon: and they came with one accord to him, and, having made Blastus the king's chamberlain their friend, they asked for peace, because their country was fed from the king's country.
21 And upon a set day Herod arrayed himself in royal apparel, and sat on the throne, and made an oration unto them.
22 And the people shouted, saying, The voice of a god, and not of a man.

23 And immediately an angel of the Lord smote him, because he gave not God the glory: and he was eaten of worms, and gave up the ghost.

1 Corinthians 1:26-29

26 For behold your calling, brethren, that not many wise after the flesh, not many mighty, not many noble, are called:
27 but God chose the foolish things of the world, that he might put to shame them that are wise; and God chose the weak things of the world, that he might put to shame the things that are strong;
28 and the base things of the world, and the things that are despised, did God choose, yea and the things that are not, that he might bring to nought the things that are:
29 that no flesh should glory before God.

Galatians 6:4

4 But let each man prove his own work, and then shall he have his glorying in regard of himself alone, and not of his neighbor.

1 Peter 5:5-6

5 Likewise, ye younger, be subject unto the elder. Yea, all of you gird yourselves with humility, to serve one another: for God resisteth the proud, but giveth grace to the humble.
6 Humble yourselves therefore under the mighty hand of God, that he may exalt you in due time;

1 John 2:16

16 For all that is in the world, the lust of the flesh and the lust of the eyes and the vain glory of life, is not of the Father, but is of the world.

Relationships and Life: Solomon's Wisdom

Wouldn't it be nice to get along better with all sorts of people in different situations? How would you like a happier marriage? Or more success in your job or business? Pray with the scripture verses from Proverbs on the following pages to improve your relationships with others. And when you feel like curling up with a good book, read the entire book of Proverbs.

 Remember!
When praying scripture, give Jesus permission to search for lies and unbelief and replace them with God's truth.

Proverbs 1:7   Key Verse
7 The fear of Jehovah is the beginning of knowledge; But the foolish despise wisdom and instruction.

Proverbs 10:12   Key Verse
12 Hatred stirreth up strifes; But love covereth all transgressions.

Proverbs 15:4   Key Verse
4 A gentle tongue is a tree of life; But perverseness therein is a breaking of the spirit.

Proverbs 16:32   Key Verse
32 He that is slow to anger is better than the mighty; And he that ruleth his spirit, than he that taketh a city.

Proverbs 1:19
19 So are the ways of every one that is greedy of gain; It taketh away the life of the owners thereof.

Proverbs 1:22
22 How long, ye simple ones, will ye love simplicity? And scoffers delight them in scoffing, And fools hate knowledge?

Proverbs 3:5-6
5 Trust in Jehovah with all thy heart, And lean not upon thine own understanding:
6 In all thy ways acknowledge him, And he will direct thy paths.

Proverbs 10:17-19
17 He is in the way of life that heedeth correction; But he that forsaketh reproof erreth.
18 He that hideth hatred is of lying lips; And he that uttereth a slander is a fool.
19 In the multitude of words there wanteth not transgression; But he that refraineth his lips doeth wisely.

Proverbs 10:21
21 The lips of the righteous feed many; But the foolish die for lack of understanding.

Proverbs 10:31
31 The mouth of the righteous bringeth forth wisdom; But the perverse tongue shall be cut off.

Proverbs 11:2
2 When pride cometh, then cometh shame; But with the lowly is wisdom.

Proverbs 11:14
14 Where no wise guidance is, the people falleth; But in the multitude of counsellors there is safety.

Proverbs 11:24-25
24 There is that scattereth, and increaseth yet more; And there is that withholdeth more than is meet, but it tendeth only to want. 25 The liberal soul shall be made fat; And he that watereth shall be watered also himself.

Proverbs 12:1
1 Whoso loveth correction loveth knowledge; But he that hateth reproof is brutish.

Proverbs 12:18
18 There is that speaketh rashly like the piercings of a sword; But the tongue of the wise is health.

Proverbs 12:24
24 The hand of the diligent shall bear rule; But the slothful shall be put under taskwork.

Proverbs 13:4
4 The soul of the sluggard desireth, and hath nothing; But the soul of the diligent shall be made fat.

Proverbs 13:10
10 By pride cometh only contention; But with the well-advised is wisdom.

Proverbs 13:11
11 Wealth gotten by vanity shall be diminished; But he that gathereth by labor shall have increase.

Proverbs 13:12
12 Hope deferred maketh the heart sick; But when the desire cometh, it is a tree of life.

Proverbs 13:18
18 Poverty and shame shall be to him that refuseth correction; But he that regardeth reproof shall be honored.

Proverbs 13:20
20 Walk with wise men, and thou shalt be wise; But the companion of fools shall smart for it.

Proverbs 14:7
7 Go into the presence of a foolish man, And thou shalt not perceive in him the lips of knowledge.

Proverbs 14:12
12 There is a way which seemeth right unto a man; But the end thereof are the ways of death.

Proverbs 14:15
15 The simple believeth every word; But the prudent man looketh well to his going.

Proverbs 14:17
17 He that is soon angry will deal foolishly; And a man of wicked devices is hated.

Proverbs 14:18
18 The simple inherit folly; But the prudent are crowned with knowledge.
Proverbs 14:23
23 In all labor there is profit; But the talk of the lips tendeth only to

penury.

Proverbs 14:26
26 In the fear of Jehovah is strong confidence; And his children shall have a place of refuge.

Proverbs 14:27
27 The fear of Jehovah is a fountain of life, That one may depart from the snares of death.

Proverbs 15:1
1 A soft answer turneth away wrath; But a grievous word stirreth up anger.

Proverbs 15:2
2 The tongue of the wise uttereth knowledge aright; But the mouth of fools poureth out folly.

Proverbs 15:8
8 The sacrifice of the wicked is an abomination to Jehovah; But the prayer of the upright is his delight.

Proverbs 15:19
19 The way of the sluggard is as a hedge of thorns; But the path of the upright is made a highway.

Proverbs 15:22
22 Where there is no counsel, purposes are disappointed; But in the multitude of counsellors they are established.

Proverbs 15:23
23 A man hath joy in the answer of his mouth; And a word in due season, how good is it!

Proverbs 15:25
25 Jehovah will root up the house of the proud; But he will establish

the border of the widow.

Proverbs 15:32-33
32 He that refuseth correction despiseth his own soul; But he that hearkeneth to reproof getteth understanding.
33 The fear of Jehovah is the instruction of wisdom; And before honor goeth humility.

Proverbs 16:9
9 A man's heart deviseth his way; But Jehovah directeth his steps.

Proverbs 16:16
16 How much better is it to get wisdom than gold! Yea, to get understanding is rather to be chosen than silver.

Proverbs 16:18
18 Pride goeth before destruction, And a haughty spirit before a fall.

Proverbs 16:23
23 The heart of the wise instructeth his mouth, And addeth learning to his lips.

Proverbs 17:3
3 The refining pot is for silver, and the furnace for gold; But Jehovah trieth the hearts.

Proverbs 18:2
2 A fool hath no delight in understanding, But only that his heart may reveal itself.

Proverbs 18:13
13 He that giveth answer before he heareth, It is folly and shame unto him.

Proverbs 18:14
14 The spirit of a man will sustain his infirmity; But a broken spirit who can bear?

Proverbs 18:19
19 A brother offended is harder to be won than a strong city; And such contentions are like the bars of a castle.

Proverbs 18:21
21 Death and life are in the power of the tongue; And they that love it shall eat the fruit thereof.

Proverbs 19:1
1 Better is the poor that walketh in his integrity Than he that is perverse in his lips and is a fool.

Proverbs 20:4
4 The sluggard will not plow by reason of the winter; Therefore he shall beg in harvest, and have nothing.

Proverbs 20:11
11 Even a child maketh himself known by his doings, Whether his work be pure, and whether it be right.

Proverbs 20:18
18 Every purpose is established by counsel; And by wise guidance make thou war.

Proverbs 20:19
19 He that goeth about as a tale-bearer revealeth secrets; Therefore company not with him that openeth wide his lips.

Proverbs 21:2
2 Every way of a man is right in his own eyes; But Jehovah weigheth the hearts.

Proverbs 21:5
5 The thoughts of the diligent tend only to plenteousness; But every one that is hasty hasteth only to want.

Proverbs 21:14
14 A gift in secret pacifieth anger; And a present in the bosom, strong wrath.

Proverbs 21:26
26 There is that coveteth greedily all the day long; But the righteous giveth and withholdeth not.

Proverbs 22:3
3 A prudent man seeth the evil, and hideth himself; But the simple pass on, and suffer for it.

Proverbs 22:11
11 He that loveth pureness of heart, For the grace of his lips the king will be his friend.

Proverbs 22:24
24 Make no friendship with a man that is given to anger; And with a wrathful man thou shalt not go:

Proverbs 22:29
29 Seest thou a man diligent in his business? he shall stand before kings; He shall not stand before mean men.

Proverbs 23:4-5
4 Weary not thyself to be rich; Cease from thine own wisdom.
5 Wilt thou set thine eyes upon that which is not? For riches certainly make themselves wings, Like an eagle that flieth toward heaven.

Proverbs 23:7
7 For as he thinketh within himself, so is he: Eat and drink, saith he to thee; But his heart is not with thee.

Proverbs 23:9
9 Speak not in the hearing of a fool; For he will despise the wisdom of thy words.

Proverbs 24:17
17 Rejoice not when thine enemy falleth, And let not thy heart be glad when he is overthrown;

Proverbs 24:29
29 Say not, I will do so to him as he hath done to me; I will render to the man according to his work.

Proverbs 25:9
9 Debate thy cause with thy neighbor himself, And disclose not the secret of another;

Proverbs 25:10
10 Lest he that heareth it revile thee, And thine infamy turn not away.

Proverbs 25:11
11 A word fitly spoken Is like apples of gold in network of silver.

Proverbs 26:17
17 He that passeth by, and vexeth himself with strife belonging not to him, Is like one that taketh a dog by the ears.

Proverbs 26:27
27 Whoso diggeth a pit shall fall therein; And he that rolleth a stone, it shall return upon him.

Proverbs 26:28
28 A lying tongue hateth those whom it hath wounded; And a flattering mouth worketh ruin.

Proverbs 27:4
4 Wrath is cruel, and anger is overwhelming; But who is able to stand before jealousy?

Proverbs 27:5
5 Better is open rebuke Than love that is hidden.

Proverbs 27:6
6 Faithful are the wounds of a friend; But the kisses of an enemy are profuse.

Proverbs 28:1
1 The wicked flee when no man pursueth; But the righteous are bold as a lion.

Proverbs 28:17
17 A man that is laden with the blood of any person Shall flee unto the pit; Let no man stay him.

Proverbs 28:19
19 He that tilleth his land shall have plenty of bread; But he that followeth after vain persons shall have poverty enough.

Proverbs 28:22
22 he that hath an evil eye hasteth after riches, And knoweth not that want shall come upon him.

Proverbs 28:26
26 He that trusteth in his own heart is a fool; But whoso walketh wisely, he shall be delivered.

Proverbs 29:1
1 He that being often reproved hardeneth his neck Shall suddenly be destroyed, and that without remedy.

Proverbs 29:19
19 A servant will not be corrected by words; For though he understand, he will not give heed.

Proverbs 29:22
22 An angry man stirreth up strife, And a wrathful man aboundeth in transgression.

Proverbs 29:26
26 Many seek the ruler's favor; But a man's judgment cometh from Jehovah.

Sorrow, Sadness, and Grief

When we lose someone close to us, it is natural to feel grief. However, if debilitating grief continues for years, it is not what Jesus would want for us. He is the lifter of our heads. He will help us deal with our grief, no doubt about it. Many times what we feel may not be grief alone, but also guilt, shame, regret, or any number of other emotions. Ask Jesus to help you define what you are feeling.

We can grieve for things other than the death of a loved one as well. Loss of a body part, such as a breast, leg, or internal organ can result in grief.

We may not realize that sadness and sorrow are also grief. Children can suffer sadness because of the loss of a parent, not only through death but divorce. Many children today are grieving the loss of a father they never knew. Although plenty of people in our culture say children are resilient and will be fine under these circumstances, I wouldn't bet my salvation on that. I believe many more children than we think are in need of Jesus' healing touch and truth.

God brings order to our lives, so when we are not living according to God's will, we are inviting disorder. Depression is another huge problem in our culture. Living with sorrow on a daily basis is what many people do. Our sorrow may be from things we've lost or greatly desired and never had. If material items are causing you sorrow, it's likely you have a wrong set of priorities. Seek to build your faith and trust in God—make Him your top priority.

> *God brings order to our lives, so when we are not living according to God's will, we are inviting disorder.*

Remember!
When praying scripture, give Jesus permission to search for lies and unbelief and replace them with God's truth.

Isaiah 53:4-5   Key Verse
4 Surely he hath borne our griefs, and carried our sorrows; yet we did esteem him stricken, smitten of God, and afflicted.
5 But he was wounded for our transgressions, he was bruised for our iniquities; the chastisement of our peace was upon him; and with his stripes we are healed.

John 16:6-7   Key Verse
6 But because I have spoken these things unto you, sorrow hath filled your heart.
7 Nevertheless I tell you the truth: It is expedient for you that I go away; for if I go not away, the Comforter will not come unto you; but if I go, I will send him unto you.

Psalms 28:7   Key Verse

7 Jehovah is my strength and my shield; My heart hath trusted in him, and I am helped: Therefore my heart greatly rejoiceth; And with my song will I praise him.

Psalms 86:4   Key Verse

4 Rejoice the soul of thy servant; For unto thee, O Lord, do I lift up my soul.

Psalms 4:7

7 Thou hast put gladness in my heart, More than they have when their grain and their new wine are increased.

Psalms 13:1-6

1 How long, O Jehovah? wilt thou forget me for ever? How long wilt thou hide thy face from me?
2 How long shall I take counsel in my soul, Having sorrow in my heart all the day? How long shall mine enemy be exalted over me?
3 Consider and answer me, O Jehovah my God: Lighten mine eyes, lest I sleep the sleep of death;
4 Lest mine enemy say, I have prevailed against him; Lest mine adversaries rejoice when I am moved.
5 But I have trusted in thy lovingkindness; My heart shall rejoice in thy salvation.
6 I will sing unto Jehovah, Because he hath dealt bountifully with me.

Psalms 16:4

4 Their sorrows shall be multiplied that give gifts for another god: Their drink-offerings of blood will I not offer, Nor take their names upon my lips.

Psalms 16:8-11

8 I have set Jehovah always before me: Because he is at my right hand, I shall not be moved.
9 Therefore my heart is glad, and my glory rejoiceth; My flesh also

shall dwell in safety.
10 For thou wilt not leave my soul to Sheol; Neither wilt thou suffer thy holy one to see corruption.
11 Thou wilt show me the path of life: In thy presence is fulness of joy; In thy right hand there are pleasures for evermore.

Psalms 30:11
11 Thou hast turned for me my mourning into dancing; Thou hast loosed my sackcloth, and girded me with gladness;

Psalms 37:3
3 Trust in Jehovah, and do good; Dwell in the land, and feed on his faithfulness.

Psalms 116:3-7
3 The cords of death compassed me, And the pains of Sheol gat hold upon me: I found trouble and sorrow.
4 Then called I upon the name of Jehovah: O Jehovah, I beseech thee, deliver my soul.
5 Gracious is Jehovah, and righteous; Yea, our God is merciful.
6 Jehovah preserveth the simple: I was brought low, and he saved me.
7 Return unto thy rest, O my soul; For Jehovah hath dealt bountifully with thee.

Ecclesiastes 11:10
10 Therefore remove sorrow from thy heart, and put away evil from thy flesh; for youth and the dawn of life are vanity.

Isaiah 35:10
10 and the ransomed of Jehovah shall return, and come with singing unto Zion; and everlasting joy shall be upon their heads: they shall obtain gladness and joy, and sorrow and sighing shall flee away.

Isaiah 51:11
11 And the ransomed of Jehovah shall return, and come with singing

unto Zion; and everlasting joy shall be upon their heads: they shall obtain gladness and joy; and sorrow and sighing shall flee away.

Isaiah 54:6
6 For Jehovah hath called thee as a wife forsaken and grieved in spirit, even a wife of youth, when she is cast off, saith thy God.

Isaiah 55:12
12 For ye shall go out with joy, and be led forth with peace: the mountains and the hills shall break forth before you into singing; and all the trees of the fields shall clap their hands.

Isaiah 61:3
3 to appoint unto them that mourn in Zion, to give unto them a garland for ashes, the oil of joy for mourning, the garment of praise for the spirit of heaviness; that they may be called trees of righteousness, the planting of Jehovah, that he may be glorified.
Jeremiah 31:13
13 Then shall the virgin rejoice in the dance, and the young men and the old together; for I will turn their mourning into joy, and will comfort them, and make them rejoice from their sorrow.

Jeremiah 31:13
13 Then shall the virgin rejoice in the dance, and the young men and the old together; for I will turn their mourning into joy, and will comfort them, and make them rejoice from their sorrow.

Lamentations 3:3
3 Surely against me he turneth his hand again and again all the day.

Luke 10:21
21 In that same hour he rejoiced in the Holy Spirit, and said, I thank thee, O Father, Lord of heaven and earth, that thou didst hide these things from the wise and understanding, and didst reveal them unto babes: yea, Father; for so it was well-pleasing in thy sight.

Sorrow, Sadness, and Grief

John 16:20
20 Verily, verily, I say unto you, that ye shall weep and lament, but the world shall rejoice: ye shall be sorrowful, but your sorrow shall be turned into joy.

John 20:20
20 And when he had said this, he showed unto them his hands and his side. The disciples therefore were glad, when they saw the Lord.

Romans 14:8
8 For whether we live, we live unto the Lord; or whether we die, we die unto the Lord: whether we live therefore, or die, we are the Lord's.

1 Corinthians 15:54-55
54 But when this corruptible shall have put on incorruption, and this mortal shall have put on immortality, then shall come to pass the saying that is written, Death is swallowed up in victory.
55 O death, where is thy victory? O death, where is thy sting?

2 Corinthians 7:10
10 For godly sorrow worketh repentance unto salvation, a repentance which bringeth no regret: but the sorrow of the world worketh death.
Philippians 1:21 (ASV)
21 For to me to live is Christ, and to die is gain.

Philippians 1:21
21 For to me to live is Christ, and to die is gain.

Philippians 2:27
27 for indeed he was sick nigh unto death: but God had mercy on him; and not on him only, but on me also, that I might not have sorrow upon sorrow.

Philippians 4:4
4 Rejoice in the Lord always: again I will say, Rejoice.

1 Thessalonians 4:13-17

13 But we would not have you ignorant, brethren, concerning them that fall asleep; that ye sorrow not, even as the rest, who have no hope.

14 For if we believe that Jesus died and rose again, even so them also that are fallen asleep in Jesus will God bring with him.

15 For this we say unto you by the word of the Lord, that we that are alive, that are left unto the coming of the Lord, shall in no wise precede them that are fallen asleep.

16 For the Lord himself shall descend from heaven, with a shout, with the voice of the archangel, and with the trump of God: and the dead in Christ shall rise first;

17 then we that are alive, that are left, shall together with them be caught up in the clouds, to meet the Lord in the air: and so shall we ever be with the Lord.

Colossians 1:11-12

11 strengthened with all power, according to the might of his glory, unto all patience and longsuffering with joy;

12 giving thanks unto the Father, who made us meet to be partakers of the inheritance of the saints in light;

1 Timothy 6:10

10 For the love of money is a root of all kinds of evil: which some reaching after have been led astray from the faith, and have pierced themselves through with many sorrows.

James 4:9-10

9 Be afflicted, and mourn, and weep: let your laughter be turned to mourning, and your joy to heaviness.

10 Humble yourselves in the sight of the Lord, and he shall exalt you.

1 Peter 5:7

7 casting all your anxiety upon him, because he careth for you.

Revelation 2:14

14 But I have a few things against thee, because thou hast there some that hold the teaching of Balaam, who taught Balak to cast a stumbling block before the children of Israel, to eat things sacrificed to idols, and to commit fornication.

Strength, Courage, and Discouragement

It is too hard to live on our own, yet many people do. Philippians 4:13 reads "*I can do all things through Christ which strengthens me,*" and according to 2 Samuel 22:23, "*For all his ordinances were before me; And as for his statutes, I did not depart from them.*" As you can see, God's Word is powerful, and in order to tap into this power, we must acknowledge and accept God's Word as truth.

> **Everyone who accepts Jesus Christ as their Lord can benefit from the power of the Holy Spirit; He is available to all believers.**

A second source of power God has for us comes from the Holy Spirit, who is sometimes referred to as "your helper." In Old Testament times, some who had the power of the Holy Spirit available to them included Moses, Gideon, Samuel, Samson, David, Elijah, and Elisha. Interestingly, the day Elijah was elevated to heaven, Elisha asked for a double portion of what Elijah had—the power of the Holy Spirit.

Today, everyone who accepts Jesus Christ as their Lord can benefit from the power of the Holy Spirit; He is available to all believers. It is as simple as asking your Heavenly Father (see Luke 11:11-13).

You can ask for gifts to improve your life and ask for help for specific purposes. For example, let's say someone did something very bad to you. Until you forgive them, that event will continue to adversely affect you. Although you know this, forgiveness seems too difficult and you just can't do it. Ask the Holy Spirit to help you and you will be greatly blessed.

People with addictions also need to ask for the Holy Spirit's help. Addictions are so hard to break without strength from God. If you haven't experienced the Holy Spirit's help, let God's truth from these scripture verses begin to teach you that God is a source of strength and courage.

Remember!
When praying scripture, give Jesus permission to search for lies and unbelief and replace them with God's truth.

Philippians 4:13   Key Verse
13 I can do all things in him that strengtheneth me.

1 John 4:13   Key Verse
13 hereby we know that we abide in him and he in us, because he hath given us of his Spirit.

1 Corinthians 10:13   Key Verse
13 There hath no temptation taken you but such as man can bear: but God is faithful, who will not suffer you to be tempted above that ye are able; but will with the temptation make also the way of escape, that ye may be able to endure it.

Colossians 1:11   Key Verse
11 strengthened with all power, according to the might of his glory, unto all patience and longsuffering with joy;

Exodus 15:2
2 Jehovah is my strength and song, And he is become my salvation: This is my God, and I will praise him; My father's God, and I will exalt him.

Deuteronomy 3:24
24 O Lord Jehovah, thou hast begun to show thy servant thy greatness, and thy strong hand: for what god is there in heaven or in earth, that can do according to thy works, and according to thy mighty acts?

Joshua 1:9
9 Have not I commanded thee? Be strong and of good courage; be not affrighted, neither be thou dismayed: for Jehovah thy God is with thee whithersoever thou goest.

2 Samuel 22:33
33 God is my strong fortress; And he guideth the perfect in his way.

1 Chronicles 16:27
27 Honor and majesty are before him: Strength and gladness are in his place.

1 Chronicles 29:12
12 Both riches and honor come of thee, and thou rulest over all; and in thy hand is power and might; and in thy hand it is to make great, and to give strength unto all.

2 Chronicles 16:9
9 For the eyes of Jehovah run to and fro throughout the whole earth, to show himself strong in the behalf of them whose heart is perfect toward him. Herein thou hast done foolishly; for from henceforth

thou shalt have wars.

Psalms 18:2
2 Jehovah is my rock, and my fortress, and my deliverer; My God, my rock, in whom I will take refuge; My shield, and the horn of my salvation, my high tower.

Psalms 21:13
13 Be thou exalted, O Jehovah, in thy strength: So will we sing and praise thy power.

Psalms 28:7
7 Jehovah is my strength and my shield; My heart hath trusted in him, and I am helped: Therefore my heart greatly rejoiceth; And with my song will I praise him.

Psalms 37:39
39 But the salvation of the righteous is of Jehovah; He is their stronghold in the time of trouble.

Psalms 46:1-2
1 God is our refuge and strength, A very present help in trouble.
2 Therefore will we not fear, though the earth do change, And though the mountains be
  shaken into the heart of the seas;

Psalms 59:17
17 Unto thee, O my strength, will I sing praises: For God is my high tower, the God of my mercy.

Psalms 71:1-3
1 In thee, O Jehovah, do I take refuge: Let me never be put to shame.
2 Deliver me in thy righteousness, and rescue me: Bow down thine ear unto me, and save me. 3 Be thou to me a rock of habitation, whereunto I may continually resort: Thou hast given commandment

to save me; For thou art my rock and my fortress.

Psalms 105:4-5

*4 Seek ye Jehovah and his strength; Seek his face evermore.
5 Remember his marvellous works that he hath done, His wonders, and the judgments of his mouth,*

Psalms 138:7

7 Though I walk in the midst of trouble, thou wilt revive me; Thou wilt stretch forth thy hand against the wrath of mine enemies, And thy right hand will save me.

Isaiah 10:27

27 And it shall come to pass in that day, that his burden shall depart from off thy shoulder, and his yoke from off thy neck, and the yoke shall be destroyed by reason of fatness.

Isaiah 35:3

3 Strengthen ye the weak hands, and confirm the feeble knees.

Isaiah 40:29-31

*29 He giveth power to the faint; and to him that hath no might he increaseth strength.
30 Even the youths shall faint and be weary, and the young men shall utterly fall:
31 but they that wait for Jehovah shall renew their strength; they shall mount up with wings as eagles; they shall run, and not be weary; they shall walk, and not faint.*

Isaiah 43:1-2

1 But now thus saith Jehovah that created thee, O Jacob, and he that formed thee, O Israel: Fear not, for I have redeemed thee; I have called thee by thy name, thou art mine. 2 When thou passest through the waters, I will be with thee; and through the rivers, they shall not overflow thee: when thou walkest through the fire, thou shalt not be burned, neither shall the flame kindle upon thee.

Daniel 11:32

32 And such as do wickedly against the covenant shall he pervert by flatteries; but the people that know their God shall be strong, and do exploits.

Joel 3:10

10 Beat your plowshares into swords, and your pruning-hooks into spears: let the weak say, I am strong.

Habakkuk 3:19

19 Jehovah, the Lord, is my strength; And he maketh my feet like hinds' feet, And will make me to walk upon my high places.

Luke 22:32

32 but I made supplication for thee, that thy faith fail not; and do thou, when once thou hast turned again, establish thy brethren.

John 15:4-5

4 Abide in me, and I in you. As the branch cannot bear fruit of itself, except it abide in the vine; so neither can ye, except ye abide in me. 5 I am the vine, ye are the branches: He that abideth in me, and I in him, the same beareth much fruit: for apart from me ye can do nothing.

Romans 8:5-6

5 For they that are after the flesh mind the things of the flesh; but they that are after the Spirit the things of the Spirit.
6 For the mind of the flesh is death; but the mind of the Spirit is life and peace:

1 Corinthians 4:20

20 For the kingdom of God is not in word, but in power

2 Corinthians 12:8-10

8 Concerning this thing I besought the Lord thrice, that it might depart from me.

9 And he hath said unto me, My grace is sufficient for thee: for my power is made perfect in weakness. Most gladly therefore will I rather glory in my weaknesses, that the power of Christ may rest upon me. 10 Wherefore I take pleasure in weaknesses, in injuries, in necessities, in persecutions, in distresses, for Christ's sake: for when I am weak, then am I strong.

Galatians 2:20
20 I have been crucified with Christ; and it is no longer I that live, but Christ living in me: and that life which I now live in the flesh I live in faith, the faith which is in the Son of God, who loved me, and gave himself up for me.

Galatians 4:7
7 So that thou art no longer a bondservant, but a son; and if a son, then an heir through God.

Galatians 5:17-18
17 For the flesh lusteth against the Spirit, and the Spirit against the flesh; for these are contrary the one to the other; that ye may not do the things that ye would. 18 But if ye are led by the Spirit, ye are not under the law.

Ephesians 3:14-21
14 For this cause I bow my knees unto the Father,
15 from whom every family in heaven and on earth is named,
16 that he would grant you, according to the riches of his glory, that ye may be strengthened with power through his Spirit in the inward man;
17 that Christ may dwell in your hearts through faith; to the end that ye, being rooted and grounded in love,
18 may be strong to apprehend with all the saints what is the breadth and length and height and depth,
19 and to know the love of Christ which passeth knowledge, that ye may be filled unto all the fullness of God.
20 Now unto him that is able to do exceeding abundantly above all

that we ask or think, according to the power that worketh in us,
21 unto him be the glory in the church and in Christ Jesus unto all generations for ever and ever. Amen.

Philippians 1:9-11
9 And this I pray, that your love may abound yet more and more in knowledge and all discernment;
10 so that ye may approve the things that are excellent; that ye may be sincere and void of offence unto the day of Christ;
11 being filled with the fruits of righteousness, which are through Jesus Christ, unto the glory and praise of God.

Philippians 2:12-13
12 So then, my beloved, even as ye have always obeyed, not as in my presence only, but now much more in my absence, work out your own salvation with fear and trembling;
13 for it is God who worketh in you both to will and to work, for his good pleasure.

Philippians 3:3
3 for we are the circumcision, who worship by the Spirit of God, and glory in Christ Jesus, and have no confidence in the flesh:

Colossians 2:14-15
14 having blotted out the bond written in ordinances that was against us, which was contrary to us: and he hath taken it out that way, nailing it to the cross;
15 having despoiled the principalities and the powers, he made a show of them openly, triumphing over them in it.

Colossians 2:9-10
9 for in him dwelleth all the fullness of the Godhead bodily,
10 and in him ye are made full, who is the head of all principality and power:

1 Thessalonians 5:23

23 And the God of peace himself sanctify you wholly; and may your spirit and soul and body be preserved entire, without blame at the coming of our Lord Jesus Christ.

1 John 2:27

27 And as for you, the anointing which ye received of him abideth in you, and ye need not that any one teach you; but as his anointing teacheth you; concerning all things, and is true, and is no lie, and even as it taught you, ye abide in him.

Jude 1:24-25

24 Now unto him that is able to guard you from stumbling, and to set you before the presence of his glory without blemish in exceeding joy,
25 to the only God our Saviour, through Jesus Christ our Lord, be glory, majesty, dominion and power, before all time, and now, and for evermore. Amen.

Taking All Thoughts Captive

Negative thoughts can be very destructive. Just thinking negatively about something you are about to do can take you down the path of failure. There are three sources for our thoughts: us, Satan, and God. While Satan screams at us, God's voice is quiet. If we don't control our own thoughts and the thoughts propagated by Satan, we will have a difficult time hearing God.

> *If we don't control our own thoughts, and the thoughts propagated by Satan, then we will have a difficult time hearing God.*

Repetitive action helps us to get things done with less effort, whether these actions are good for us or not. By the same token, repetitive thoughts make it more likely we will follow through on what we are thinking about. When thoughts are negative or unwholesome, that is a path which can lead toward destruction.

> **Remember!**
> When praying scripture, give Jesus permission to search for lies and unbelief and replace them with God's truth.

2 Corinthians 10:4-5   Key Verse
4 (for the weapons of our warfare are not of the flesh, but mighty before God to the casting down of strongholds),
5 casting down imaginations, and every high thing that is exalted against the knowledge of God, and bringing every thought into captivity to the obedience of Christ;

Isaiah 26:3   Key Verse
3 Thou wilt keep him in perfect peace, whose mind is stayed on thee; because he trusteth in thee.

Mark 13:5   Key Verse
5 And Jesus began to say unto them, Take heed that no man lead you astray.

Jeremiah 29:11   Key Verse
11 For I know the thoughts that I think toward you, saith Jehovah, thoughts of peace, and not of evil, to give you hope in your latter end.

Proverbs 12:5
5 The thoughts of the righteous are just; But the counsels of the wicked are deceit.

Proverbs 15:26
26 Evil devices are an abomination to Jehovah; But pleasant words are pure.

Proverbs 16:20

20 He that giveth heed unto the word shall find good; And whoso trusteth in Jehovah, happy is he.

Proverbs 18:21

21 Death and life are in the power of the tongue; And they that love it shall eat the fruit thereof.

Proverbs 23:7

7 For as he thinketh within himself, so is he: Eat and drink, saith he to thee; But his heart is not with thee.

Matthew 12:34

34 Ye offspring of vipers, how can ye, being evil, speak good things? for out of the abundance of the heart the mouth speaketh.

Matthew 15:19-20

19 For out of the heart come forth evil thoughts, murders, adulteries, fornications, thefts, false witness, railings:
20 these are the things which defile the man; but to eat with unwashen hands defileth not the man.

Mark 7:15

15 there is nothing from without the man, that going into him can defile him; but the things which proceed out of the man are those that defile the man.

Mark 7:18-23

18 And he saith unto them, Are ye so without understanding also? Perceive ye not, that whatsoever from without goeth into the man, it cannot defile him;
19 because it goeth not into his heart, but into his belly, and goeth out into the draught? This he said, making all meats clean.
20 And he said, That which proceedeth out of the man, that defileth the man.
21 For from within, out of the heart of men, evil thoughts proceed,

fornications, thefts, murders, adulteries,
22 covetings, wickednesses, deceit, lasciviousness, an evil eye, railing, pride, foolishness:
23 all these evil things proceed from within, and defile the man.

John 16:13-15
13 Howbeit when he, the Spirit of truth, is come, he shall guide you into all the truth: for he shall not speak from himself; but what things soever he shall hear, these shall he speak: and he shall declare unto you the things that are to come.
14 He shall glorify me: for he shall take of mine, and shall declare it unto you.
15 All things whatsoever the Father hath are mine: therefore said I, that he taketh of mine, and shall declare it unto you.

Romans 12:2
2 And be not fashioned according to this world: but be ye transformed by the renewing of your mind, and ye may prove what is the good and acceptable and perfect will of God.

1 Corinthians 3:18-23
18 Let no man deceive himself. If any man thinketh that he is wise among you in this world, let him become a fool, that he may become wise.
19 For the wisdom of this world is foolishness with God. For it is written, He that taketh the wise in their craftiness:
20 and again, The Lord knoweth the reasonings of the wise that they are vain.
21 Wherefore let no one glory in men. For all things are yours;
22 whether Paul, or Apollos, or Cephas, or the world, or life, or death, or things present, or things to come; all are yours;
23 and ye are Christ's; and Christ is God's.

1 Corinthians 10:12
12 Wherefore let him that thinketh he standeth take heed lest he fall.

2 Corinthians 4:13-14

13 But having the same spirit of faith, according to that which is written, I believed, and therefore did I speak; we also believe, and therefore also we speak;
14 knowing that he that raised up the Lord Jesus shall raise up us also with Jesus, and shall present us with you.

Ephesians 4:22-24

22 that ye put away, as concerning your former manner of life, the old man, that waxeth corrupt after the lusts of deceit;
23 and that ye be renewed in the spirit of your mind,
24 and put on the new man, that after God hath been created in righteousness and holiness of truth.

Ephesians 6:10-18

10 Finally, be strong in the Lord, and in the strength of his might.
11 Put on the whole armor of God, that ye may be able to stand against the wiles of the devil.
12 For our wrestling is not against flesh and blood, but against the principalities, against the powers, against the world-rulers of this darkness, against the spiritual hosts of wickedness in the heavenly places.
13 Wherefore take up the whole armor of God, that ye may be able to withstand in the evil day, and, having done all, to stand.
14 Stand therefore, having girded your loins with truth, and having put on the breastplate of righteousness,
15 and having shod your feet with the preparation of the gospel of peace;
16 withal taking up the shield of faith, wherewith ye shall be able to quench all the fiery darts of the evil one.
17 And take the helmet of salvation, and the sword of the Spirit, which is the word of God:
18 with all prayer and supplication praying at all seasons in the Spirit, and watching thereunto in all perseverance and supplication for all the saints,

Philippians 2:5
5 Have this mind in you, which was also in Christ Jesus:

Philippians 4:8
8 Finally, brethren, whatsoever things are true, whatsoever things are honorable, whatsoever things are just, whatsoever things are pure, whatsoever things are lovely, whatsoever things are of good report; if there be any virtue, and if there be any praise, think on these things.

Colossians 2:20-23
20 If ye died with Christ from the rudiments of the world, why, as though living in the world, do ye subject yourselves to ordinances,
21 Handle not, nor taste, nor touch
22 (all which things are to perish with the using), after the precepts and doctrines of men?
23 Which things have indeed a show of wisdom in will-worship, and humility, and severity to the body; but are not of any value against the indulgence of the flesh.

Colossians 3:1-4
1 If then ye were raised together with Christ, seek the things that are above, where Christ is, seated on the right hand of God.
2 Set your mind on the things that are above, not on the things that are upon the earth.
3 For ye died, and your life is hid with Christ in God.
4 When Christ, who is our life, shall be manifested, then shall ye also with him be manifested in glory.

James 2:19
19 Thou believest that God is one; thou doest well: the demons also believe, and shudder.

1 John 2:15-17
15 Love not the world, neither the things that are in the world. If any man love the world, the love of the Father is not in him.

16 For all that is in the world, the lust of the flesh and the lust of the eyes and the vain glory of life, is not of the Father, but is of the world.

17 And the world passeth away, and the lust thereof: but he that doeth the will of God abideth for ever.

TRUST

"He shall not be afraid of evil tidings: His heart is fixed, trusting in Jehovah (Psalms 112:7)."

Does that sound like you? How about this verse?

" ... knowing that he that raised up the Lord Jesus shall raise up us also with Jesus, and shall present us with you (2 Corinthians 4:14)."

Are these scripture verses consistent with how you are living your life? For most of us, probably not. We worry about even the smallest things. Fear steals our peace, we lack hope, and we are missing contentment.

Trusting doesn't mean that we shouldn't seek medical attention for our health problems, but do we ask God for His help? For some people, medical science has become an idol. Yet within the medical community we see that new age healing has become an alternative because medical science doesn't have all of the answers. So, do you ask for God's healing before and while receiving medical attention, or only after, as a last resort?

Your life can be stressful if you are not trusting God. Think of all the energy you would save by not worrying. Trust is the positive force we need to develop in our lives as an antidote to fear and hopelessness. You will see that as you break free from fear, you will trust more. And as you trust more, fear will have less of a grip on you. It's never simple. You can't break it down into one easy formula or one life-changing book. Life is complex and our adversary certainly knows this.

> *Think of all the energy you would save by not worrying.*

Remember!
When praying scripture, give Jesus permission to search for lies and unbelief and replace them with God's truth.

Matthew 6:31-34   Key Verse
31 Be not therefore anxious, saying, What shall we eat? or, What shall we drink? or, Wherewithal shall we be clothed?
32 For after all these things do the Gentiles seek; for your heavenly Father knoweth that ye have need of all these things.
33 But seek ye first his kingdom, and his righteousness; and all these things shall be added unto you.
34 Be not therefore anxious for the morrow: for the morrow will be anxious for itself. Sufficient unto the day is the evil thereof.

John 10:10   Key Verse
10 The thief cometh not, but that he may steal, and kill, and destroy: I came that they may have life, and may have it abundantly.

Psalms 9:10   Key Verse
10 And they that know thy name will put their trust in thee; For thou, Jehovah, hast not forsaken them that seek thee.

Jude 1:24-25   Key Verse
24 Now unto him that is able to guard you from stumbling, and to set you before the presence of his glory without blemish in exceeding joy,
25 to the only God our Saviour, through Jesus Christ our Lord, be glory, majesty, dominion and power, before all time, and now, and for evermore. Amen.

Psalms 55:22   Key Verse
22 Cast thy burden upon Jehovah, and he will sustain thee: He will never suffer the righteous to be moved.

Deuteronomy 7:9
9 Know therefore that Jehovah thy God, he is God, the faithful God, who keepeth covenant and lovingkindness with them that love him and keep his commandments to a thousand generations,

Deuteronomy 7:13
13 and he will love thee, and bless thee, and multiply thee; he will also bless the fruit of thy body and the fruit of thy ground, thy grain and thy new wine and thine oil, the increase of thy cattle and the young of thy flock, in the land which he sware unto thy fathers to give thee.

Deuteronomy 32:35
35 Vengeance is mine, and recompense, At the time when their foot shall slide: For the day of their calamity is at hand, And the things that are to come upon them shall make haste.

2 Samuel 22:3
3 God, my rock, in him will I take refuge; My shield, and the horn of my salvation, my high tower, and my refuge; My saviour, thou

savest me from violence.

2 Samuel 22:31
31 As for God, his way is perfect: The word of Jehovah is tried; He is a shield unto all them that take refuge in him.

Psalms 4:5
5 Offer the sacrifices of righteousness, And put your trust in Jehovah.

Psalms 5:11
11 But let all those that take refuge in thee rejoice, Let them ever shout for joy, because thou defendest them: Let them also that love thy name be joyful in thee.

Psalms 13:5
5 But I have trusted in thy lovingkindness; My heart shall rejoice in thy salvation.

Psalms 31:1
1 In thee, O Jehovah, do I take refuge; Let me never be put to shame: Deliver me in thy righteousness.

Psalms 37:3-5
3 Trust in Jehovah, and do good; Dwell in the land, and feed on his faithfulness.
4 Delight thyself also in Jehovah; And he will give thee the desires of thy heart.
5 Commit thy way unto Jehovah; Trust also in him, and he will bring it to pass.

Psalms 40:4
4 Blessed is the man that maketh Jehovah his trust, And respecteth not the proud, nor such as turn aside to lies.

Psalms 58:10-11

10 The righteous shall rejoice when he seeth the vengeance: He shall wash his feet in the blood of the wicked;
11 So that men shall say, Verily there is a reward for the righteous: Verily there is a God that judgeth in the earth

Psalms 62:8

8 Trust in him at all times, ye people; Pour out your heart before him: God is a refuge for us. Selah

Psalms 84:11-12

11 For Jehovah God is a sun and a shield: Jehovah will give grace and glory; No good thing will he withhold from them that walk uprightly.
12 O Jehovah of hosts, Blessed is the man that trusteth in thee.

Psalms 91:3-5

3 For he will deliver thee from the snare of the fowler, And from the deadly pestilence.
4 He will cover thee with his pinions, And under his wings shalt thou take refuge: His truth is a shield and a buckler.
5 Thou shalt not be afraid for the terror by night, Nor for the arrow that flieth by day;

Psalms 100:4-5

4 Enter into his gates with thanksgiving, And into his courts with praise: Give thanks unto him, and bless his name.
5 For Jehovah is good; His lovingkindness endureth for ever, And his faithfulness unto all generations.

Psalms 103:1-5

1 Bless Jehovah, O my soul; And all that is within me, bless his holy name.
2 Bless Jehovah, O my soul, And forget not all his benefits:
3 Who forgiveth all thine iniquities; Who healeth all thy diseases;
4 Who redeemeth thy life from destruction; Who crowneth thee

with lovingkindness and tender mercies;
5 Who satisfieth thy desire with good things, So that thy youth is renewed like the eagle.

Psalms 111:5
5 He hath given food unto them that fear him: He will ever be mindful of his covenant.

Psalms 112:7
7 He shall not be afraid of evil tidings: His heart is fixed, trusting in Jehovah.

Psalms 125:1
1 They that trust in Jehovah Are as mount Zion, which cannot be moved, but abideth for ever.

Psalms 132:15
15 I will abundantly bless her provision: I will satisfy her poor with bread.

Psalms 139:9-10
9 If I take the wings of the morning, And dwell in the uttermost parts of the sea;
10 Even there shall thy hand lead me, And thy right hand shall hold me.

Psalms 145:14
14 Jehovah upholdeth all that fall, And raiseth up all those that are bowed down.

Psalms 145:18
18 Jehovah is nigh unto all them that call upon him, To all that call upon him in truth.

Psalms 147:14
14 He maketh peace in thy borders; He filleth thee with the finest of

the wheat.

Proverbs 3:5-6

5 Trust in Jehovah with all thy heart, And lean not upon thine own understanding:
6 In all thy ways acknowledge him, And he will direct thy paths.

Isaiah 26:3-4

3 Thou wilt keep him in perfect peace, whose mind is stayed on thee; because he trusteth in thee.

Isaiah 55:3

3 Incline your ear, and come unto me; hear, and your soul shall live: and I will make an everlasting covenant with you, even the sure mercies of David.
4 Trust ye in Jehovah for ever; for in Jehovah, even Jehovah, is an everlasting rock.

Isaiah 50:10

10 Who is among you that feareth Jehovah, that obeyeth the voice of his servant? he that walketh in darkness, and hath no light, let him trust in the name of Jehovah, and rely upon his God.

Jeremiah 17:5-8

5 Thus saith Jehovah: Cursed is the man that trusteth in man, and maketh flesh his arm, and whose heart departeth from Jehovah.
6 For he shall be like the heath in the desert, and shall not see when good cometh, but shall inhabit the parched places in the wilderness, a salt land and not inhabited.
7 Blessed is the man that trusteth in Jehovah, and whose trust Jehovah is.
8 For he shall be as a tree planted by the waters, that spreadeth out its roots by the river, and shall not fear when heat cometh, but its leaf shall be green; and shall not be careful in the year of drought, neither shall cease from yielding fruit.

Jeremiah 17:11
11 As the partridge that sitteth on eggs which she hath not laid, so is he that getteth riches, and not by right; in the midst of his days they shall leave him, and at his end he shall be a fool.

Daniel 6:23
23 Then was the king exceeding glad, and commanded that they should take Daniel up out of the den. So Daniel was taken up out of the den, and no manner of hurt was found upon him, because he had trusted in his God.

Matthew 6:11
11 Give us this day our daily bread.

Matthew 6:6
6 But thou, when thou prayest, enter into thine inner chamber, and having shut thy door, pray to thy Father who is in secret, and thy Father who seeth in secret shall recompense thee.

Matthew 6:26
26 Behold the birds of the heaven, that they sow not, neither do they reap, nor gather into barns; and your heavenly Father feedeth them. Are not ye of much more value then they?

Matthew 16:25
25 For whosoever would save his life shall lose it: and whosoever shall lose his life for my sake shall find it.

Mark 6:31
31 And he saith unto them, Come ye yourselves apart into a desert place, and rest a while. For there were many coming and going, and they had no leisure so much as to eat.

Luke 24:30-32
30 And it came to pass, when he had sat down with them to meat, he took the bread and blessed; and breaking it he gave to them.

31 And their eyes were opened, and they knew him; and he vanished out of their sight.
32 And they said one to another, Was not our heart burning within us, while he spake to us in the way, while he opened to us the scriptures?

John 6:35-40

35 Jesus said unto them. I am the bread of life: he that cometh to me shall not hunger, and he that believeth on me shall never thirst.
36 But I said unto you, that ye have seen me, and yet believe not.
37 All that which the Father giveth me shall come unto me; and him that cometh to me I will in no wise cast out.
38 For I am come down from heaven, not to do mine own will, but the will of him that sent me.
39 And this is the will of him that sent me, that of all that which he hath given me I should lose nothing, but should raise it up at the last day.
40 For this is the will of my Father, that every one that beholdeth the Son, and believeth on him, should have eternal life; and I will raise him up at the last day.

John 7:37-38

37 Now on the last day, the great day of the feast, Jesus stood and cried, saying, If any man thirst, let him come unto me and drink.
38 He that believeth on me, as the scripture hath said, from within him shall flow rivers of living water.

John 14:26

26 But the Comforter, even the Holy Spirit, whom the Father will send in my name, he shall teach you all things, and bring to your remembrance all that I said unto you.

Acts 2:21

21 And it shall be, that whosoever shall call on the name of the Lord shall be saved.

Romans 2:2
2 And we know that the judgment of God is according to truth against them that practice such things.

Romans 8:28-29
28 And we know that to them that love God all things work together for good, even to them that are called according to his purpose.
29 For whom he foreknew, he also foreordained to be conformed to the image of his Son, that he might be the firstborn among many brethren:

Romans 8:31-34
31 What then shall we say to these things? If God is for us, who is against us?
32 He that spared not his own Son, but delivered him up for us all, how shall he not also with him freely give us all things?
33 Who shall lay anything to the charge of God's elect? It is God that justifieth;
34 who is he that condemneth? It is Christ Jesus that died, yea rather, that was raised from the dead, who is at the right hand of God, who also maketh intercession for us.

2 Corinthians 4:13-14
13 But having the same spirit of faith, according to that which is written, I believed, and therefore did I speak; we also believe, and therefore also we speak;
14 knowing that he that raised up the Lord Jesus shall raise up us also with Jesus, and shall present us with you.

Philippians 1:29
29 because to you it hath been granted in the behalf of Christ, not only to believe on him, but also to suffer in his behalf:

Philippians 2:12-13
12 So then, my beloved, even as ye have always obeyed, not as in my presence only, but now much more in my absence, work out your

own salvation with fear and trembling;
13 for it is God who worketh in you both to will and to work, for his good pleasure.

Colossians 3:4

4 When Christ, who is our life, shall be manifested, then shall ye also with him be manifested in glory.

Colossians 2:7-10

7 rooted and builded up in him, and established in your faith, even as ye were taught, abounding in thanksgiving.
8 Take heed lest there shall be any one that maketh spoil of you through his philosophy and vain deceit, after the tradition of men, after the rudiments of the world, and not after Christ:
9 for in him dwelleth all the fullness of the Godhead bodily,
10 and in him ye are made full, who is the head of all principality and power:

2 Thessalonians 2:13-17

13 But we are bound to give thanks to God always for you, brethren beloved of the Lord, for that God chose you from the beginning unto salvation in sanctification of the Spirit and belief of the truth:
14 whereunto he called you through our gospel, to the obtaining of the glory of our Lord Jesus Christ.
15 So then, brethren, stand fast, and hold the traditions which ye were taught, whether by word, or by epistle of ours.
16 Now our Lord Jesus Christ himself, and God our Father who loved us and gave us eternal comfort and good hope through grace,
17 comfort your hearts and establish them in every good work and word.

Hebrews 4:14

14 Having then a great high priest, who hath passed through the heavens, Jesus the Son of God, let us hold fast our confession.

Hebrews 10:23
23 let us hold fast the confession of our hope that it waver not; for he is faithful that promised:

Hebrews 12:1
1 Therefore let us also, seeing we are compassed about with so great a cloud of witnesses, lay aside every weight, and the sin which doth so easily beset us, and let us run with patience the race that is set before us,

James 1:6
6 But let him ask in faith, nothing doubting: for he that doubteth is like the surge of the sea driven by the wind and tossed.

James 2:19
19 Thou believest that God is one; thou doest well: the demons also believe, and shudder.

James 4:2
2 Ye lust, and have not: ye kill, and covet, and cannot obtain: ye fight and war; ye have not, because ye ask not.

1 Peter 5:7
7 casting all your anxiety upon him, because he careth for you.

1 John 4:4
4 Ye are of God, my little children, and have overcome them: because greater is he that is in you than he that is in the world.

WORRY

Worry comes from fear. Most often we worry about future events. Worry is something we do—it's active—in contrast to experiencing stress, which can be passive. When we worry, our mind is actively engaged in thinking about things we are afraid of. This creates stress and can lead to sleep deprivation. Sometimes people play out fictitious scenarios in their mind, which adds to the worry. Instead of focusing on our fears, and worrying, we must ask Jesus (and the Holy Spirit) to help control our thoughts. We need to trust in the Lord. Turn over your worry to Jesus and not allow negative thoughts to control you.

According to 2 Corinthians 10:5, we should *"take captive every thought to the Word of God."*

If we are worrying over events within our control, we need to ask the Lord to help us accomplish what we need to do. If we are worrying about events and people which we cannot control, we need to let that go and turn it over to Jesus.

Remember!
When praying scripture, give Jesus permission to search for lies and unbelief and replace them with God's truth.

Mark 4:19   Key Verse
19 and the cares of the world, and the deceitfulness of riches, and the lusts of other things entering in, choke the word, and it becometh unfruitful.

1 Peter 5:7   Key Verse
7 casting all your anxiety upon him, because he careth for you.

Psalms 37:4
4 Delight thyself also in Jehovah; And he will give thee the desires of thy heart.

Psalms 55:22
22 Cast thy burden upon Jehovah, and he will sustain thee: He will never suffer the righteous to be moved.

Psalms 138:8
8 Jehovah will perfect that which concerneth me: Thy lovingkindness, O Jehovah, endureth for ever; Forsake not the works of thine own hands.

Matthew 6:32-34
32 For after all these things do the Gentiles seek; for your heavenly Father knoweth that ye have need of all these things.
33 But seek ye first his kingdom, and his righteousness; and all these things shall be added unto you.
34 Be not therefore anxious for the morrow: for the morrow will be anxious for itself. Sufficient unto the day is the evil thereof.

Matthew 11:28-30
28 Come unto me, all ye that labor and are heavy laden, and I will give you rest.
29 Take my yoke upon you, and learn of me; for I am meek and lowly in heart: and ye shall find rest unto your souls.
30 For my yoke is easy, and my burden is light.

Philippians 4:4
4 Rejoice in the Lord always: again I will say, Rejoice.

Philippians 4:6-7
6 In nothing be anxious; but in everything by prayer and supplication with thanksgiving let your requests be made known unto God.
7 And the peace of God, which passeth all understanding, shall guard your hearts and your thoughts in Christ Jesus.

Philippians 4:11
11 Not that I speak in respect of want: for I have learned, in whatsoever state I am, therein to be content.

Your Value, an Unloving Self-Worth, and Self-Hate

This topic is about you and what you believe about yourself. Do you hate yourself for who you are or what you have done? We have heard much about self-esteem training for children in schools. While the idea may sound good, no amount of human logic can overcome feelings of self-hate. We repress those emotions and then put a wall around them.

With the self-esteem training, it is evident we can obtain a high degree of self-centeredness and pridefulness. We may put up a strong front, which serves us most of the time on the surface. However, when we hit life's bumps, we will live what we believe. If our beliefs are based on experiences of hurt as a child, such as not receiving love or being made to feel we are worthless, then these feelings will manifest when our lives are pushed by current events. People

> *People who are self-destructive are living the experience and belief of what they perceive their value to be.*

who are self-destructive are living the experience and belief of what they perceive their value to be.

Only by allowing our negative beliefs to be reversed can our self-assessment be changed for the better. Let God's Word reverse these beliefs and transform them into the positive truth that God knows about you. You have value to God and other people. You may also find that you need to receive ministry from someone knowledgeable that can help you work through forgiveness and healing past hurts.

Remember!
When praying scripture, give Jesus permission to search for lies and unbelief and replace them with God's truth.

Ephesians 2:10   Key Verse
10 For we are his workmanship, created in Christ Jesus for good works, which God afore prepared that we should walk in them.

John 17:23   Key Verse
23 I in them, and thou in me, that they may be perfected into one; that the world may know that thou didst send me, and lovedst them, even as thou lovedst me.

Galatians 2:20   Key Verse
20 I have been crucified with Christ; and it is no longer I that live, but Christ living in me: and that life which I now live in the flesh I live in faith, the faith which is in the Son of God, who loved me, and gave himself up for me.

Jeremiah 1:5   Key Verse
5 Before I formed thee in the belly I knew thee, and before thou camest forth out of the womb I sanctified thee; I have appointed thee a prophet unto the nations.

Genesis 1:27

27 And God created man in his own image, in the image of God created he him; male and female created he them.

1 Samuel 16:7

7 But Jehovah said unto Samuel, Look not on his countenance, or on the height of his stature; because I have rejected him: for Jehovah seeth not as man seeth; for man looketh on the outward appearance, but Jehovah looketh on the heart.

Psalms 8:3-6

3 When I consider thy heavens, the work of thy fingers, The moon and the stars, which thou hast ordained;
4 What is man, that thou art mindful of him? And the son of man, that thou visitest him?
5 For thou hast made him but little lower than God, And crownest him with glory and honor.
6 Thou makest him to have dominion over the works of thy hands; Thou hast put all things under his feet:

Psalms 8:5

5 For thou hast made him but little lower than God, And crownest him with glory and honor.

Psalms 27:10

10 When my father and my mother forsake me, Then Jehovah will take me up.

Psalms 100:3-5

3 Know ye that Jehovah, he is God: It is he that hath made us, and we are his; We are his people, and the sheep of his pasture.
4 Enter into his gates with thanksgiving, And into his courts with praise: Give thanks unto him, and bless his name.
5 For Jehovah is good; His lovingkindness endureth for ever, And his faithfulness unto all generations.

Psalms 139:4

4 For there is not a word in my tongue, But, lo, O Jehovah, thou knowest it altogether.

Psalms 139:14-16

14 I will give thanks unto thee; For I am fearfully and wonderfully made: Wonderful are thy works; And that my soul knoweth right well.
15 My frame was not hidden from thee, When I was made in secret, And curiously wrought in the lowest parts of the earth.
16 Thine eyes did see mine unformed substance; And in thy book they were all written, Even the days that were ordained for me, When as yet there was none of them.

Song of Songs 7:10

10 I am my beloved's; And his desire is toward me.

Isaiah 41:9

9 thou whom I have taken hold of from the ends of the earth, and called from the corners thereof, and said unto thee, Thou art my servant, I have chosen thee and not cast thee away;

Isaiah 43:4

4 Since thou hast been precious in my sight, and honorable, and I have loved thee; therefore will I give men in thy stead, and peoples instead of thy life.

Isaiah 49:16

16 Behold, I have graven thee upon the palms of my hands; thy walls are continually before me.

Isaiah 62:5

5 For as a young man marrieth a virgin, so shall thy sons marry thee; and as the bridegroom rejoiceth over the bride, so shall thy God rejoice over thee.

Ezekiel 28:11-15

11 Moreover the word of Jehovah came unto me, saying,
12 Son of man, take up a lamentation over the king of Tyre, and say unto him, Thus saith the Lord Jehovah: Thou sealest up the sum, full of wisdom, and perfect in beauty.
13 Thou wast in Eden, the garden of God; every precious stone was thy covering, the sardius, the topaz, and the diamond, the beryl, the onyx, and the jasper, the sapphire, the emerald, and the carbuncle, and gold: the workmanship of thy tabrets and of thy pipes was in thee; in the day that thou wast created they were prepared.
14 Thou wast the anointed cherub that covereth: and I set thee, so that thou wast upon the holy mountain of God; thou hast walked up and down in the midst of the stones of fire.
15 Thou wast perfect in thy ways from the day that thou wast created, till unrighteousness was found in thee.

Zechariah 2:8

8 For thus saith Jehovah of hosts: After glory hath he sent me unto the nations which plundered you; for he that toucheth you toucheth the apple of his eye.

Matthew 6:26

26 Behold the birds of the heaven, that they sow not, neither do they reap, nor gather into barns; and your heavenly Father feedeth them. Are not ye of much more value then they?

Matthew 10:29-31

29 Are not two sparrows sold for a penny? and not one of them shall fall on the ground without your Father:
30 but the very hairs of your head are all numbered.
31 Fear not therefore: ye are of more value than many sparrows.

John 15:13

13 Greater love hath no man than this, that a man lay down his life for his friends.

John 15:16
16 Ye did not choose me, but I chose you, and appointed you, that ye should go and bear fruit, and that your fruit should abide: that whatsoever ye shall ask of the Father in my name, he may give it you.

Romans 8:31
31 What then shall we say to these things? If God is for us, who is against us?

Romans 8:34
34 who is he that condemneth? It is Christ Jesus that died, yea rather, that was raised from the dead, who is at the right hand of God, who also maketh intercession for us.

1 Corinthians 13:12
12 For now we see in a mirror, darkly; but then face to face: now I know in part; but then shall I know fully even as also I was fully known.

2 Corinthians 3:5
5 not that we are sufficient of ourselves, to account anything as from ourselves; but our sufficiency is from God;

2 Corinthians 3:18
18 But we all, with unveiled face beholding as in a mirror the glory of the Lord, are transformed into the same image from glory to glory, even as from the Lord the Spirit.

2 Corinthians 5:17
17 Wherefore if any man is in Christ, he is a new creature: the old things are passed away; behold, they are become new.

2 Corinthians 5:21
21 Him who knew no sin he made to be sin on our behalf; that we might become the righteousness of God in him.

2 Corinthians 10:7

7 Ye look at the things that are before your face. If any man trusteth in himself that he is Christ's, let him consider this again with himself, that, even as he is Christ's, so also are we.

Ephesians 2:6

6 and raised us up with him, and made us to sit with him in the heavenly places, in Christ Jesus:

Colossians 1:26-27

26 even the mystery which hath been hid for ages and generations: but now hath it been manifested to his saints,
27 to whom God was pleased to make known what is the riches of the glory of this mystery among the Gentiles, which is Christ in you, the hope of glory:

Colossians 2:6-7

6 As therefore ye received Christ Jesus the Lord, so walk in him,
7 rooted and builded up in him, and established in your faith, even as ye were taught, abounding in thanksgiving.

Colossians 3:1

1 If then ye were raised together with Christ, seek the things that are above, where Christ is, seated on the right hand of God.

Colossians 3:3

3 For ye died, and your life is hid with Christ in God.

Colossians 3:10

10 and have put on the new man, that is being renewed unto knowledge after the image of him that created him:

1 Thessalonians 5:18

18 in everything give thanks: for this is the will of God in Christ Jesus to you-ward.

2 Timothy 1:12

12 For which cause I suffer also these things: yet I am not ashamed; for I know him whom I have believed, and I am persuaded that he is able to guard that which I have committed unto him against that day.

Hebrews 13:6

6 So that with good courage we say, The Lord is my helper; I will not fear: What shall man do unto me?

James 1:17-18

17 Every good gift and every perfect gift is from above, coming down from the Father of lights, with whom can be no variation, neither shadow that is cast by turning.
18 Of his own will he brought us forth by the word of truth, that we should be a kind of firstfruits of his creatures.

1 Peter 2:9

9 But ye are a elect race, a royal priesthood, a holy nation, a people for God's own possession, that ye may show forth the excellencies of him who called you out of darkness into his marvellous light:

1 John 3:2

2 Beloved, now are we children of God, and it is not yet made manifest what we shall be. We know that, if he shall be manifested, we shall be like him; for we shall see him even as he is.

1 John 4:17-19

17 Herein is love made perfect with us, that we may have boldness in the day of judgment; because as he is, even so are we in this world.
18 There is no fear in love: but perfect love casteth out fear, because fear hath punishment; and he that feareth is not made perfect in love.
19 We love, because he first loved us.

Psalms

The following list of scripture chapters comes from the book of Psalms. The Psalms are very powerful. These Psalms lend themselves to various topics and life situations. The numbers in the left column identify chapters, while the descriptions in the right column define the subject of the particular Psalm. David wrote many of them while he was on the run from Saul, who wanted to get rid of him (because of Saul's own pride and envy). David's Psalms were written about the subjects of praying for protection, defeating enemies, overcoming sin, hearing God's instruction, and other similar topics. While our place in life is different than that of David's, our needs are similar. David didn't hold anything back; if he felt it or thought it, he shared it with God. That is why the Psalms speak to so many people—we can relate.

When conducting a meeting, using a particular Psalm can work well. If you are ministering to someone for healing or deliverance, there also may be a Psalm that speaks to what needs to be done.

Remember!
When praying scripture, give Jesus permission to search for lies and unbelief and replace them with God's truth.

Psalms
Chapter / Topic

1 Righteousness
3 Trusting God's protection and peace (overcoming fear)
5 Protection from the lies of enemies
6 Deliverance from trouble (and healing)
7 Justice from persecution and slander
8 Human value / understanding one's self
9 Thanking God for turning back enemies
10 Injustice
11 Trusting God when facing problems
12 Protection from those trying to manipulate you
13 Prayer for depression / patience
16 Joy to overcome sadness
19 What's controlling you—ask to be shown
20 Victory in battle
21 Victory after battle
23 Our guide / comfort
25 To be shown God's ways
27 God as an antidote for fear and loneliness (hope and strength)
31 Commitment to God in times of stress
32 Forgiveness for true joy

34	Trusting the Lord when you are down
35	Defeating enemies
36	God pours out His love
38	Healing and protection for confessing your sins
39	Depression /apart from God, life is fleeting and empty
40	Patience for God's message
41	Feeling forsaken
42	Depression / thirsting for God
43	Courage
46	Refuge / serenity / peace from fear
51	Pleas for mercy / forgiveness / cleansing
55	When friends hurt us
56	Trusting God in the midst of fear
57	Protection
58	God's justice
59	God's love is our place of safety
62	God is our sanctuary
63	Depression / a desire for God's presence and provision
67	Joy from spreading the Good News
70	Hasty prayer for help
76	Requesting God punish evil-doers
78	Trust in God now
91	Spiritual warfare /God's protection
93	A reminder of God's great power
100	Thanksgiving
101	Integrity in our life requires
102	Cure for distress

- 103 God's great love for us
- 136 God's endless love
- 137 Life's regrets and sorrow
- 138 The Lord working in your life
- 139 Worthiness and permission for God to work in your life
- 140 Deliverance (concentrating on your future life with God)
- 141 Prayer for overcoming temptation
- 142 Prayer when overwhelmed
- 143 Prayer for hopelessness and depression
- 145 Trust
- 145 Healing

DISEASE APPENDIX

The list that follows presents diseases and their related emotional issues, which are suggested topics you should consider when beginning to direct your prayers. Yet don't be too rigid in your thinking because each person has unique circumstances. Remember, while reading or praying with scripture verses under a certain topic you may perhaps be drawn to another topic. If you have a number of ailments, you will see considerable overlap.

Personally, I have seen diseases healed by praying with scripture verses; it may be all you need to do. However, you might also need to heal deep emotional wounds, and/or allow time for the Holy Spirit to help grow your faith. In addition, many times it seems that Jesus heals us in layers, possibly because He knows we can handle only so much at a time, or so that it can be revealed to us how much He is working in our lives. We should glorify Him for each step of our healing!

As already mentioned, you may well need to have Jesus search your life and show you things you need to deal with further. At times, we miss what the Holy Spirit is trying to tell us. Our discernment possibly will need to improve. Returning to scripture will help to lead us further along. And you possibly will find that when your negative strongholds are weakened, the prayers of concerned friends will be much more effective.

Many of us cannot see any connection between our spiritual condition and disease. Because it is widely taught that God doesn't punish people here on earth, some might interpret it to mean that a person's actions do not affect their life on the planet. While I believe that God doesn't punish us now, He does chastise or correct those whom He loves. I do believe when we live outside of God's will (as shown in the Bible) there is a separation, or wall, between us and God, which interferes with us receiving God's blessings. Protection and healing are two of His blessings. So when we live outside of God's will, we are on our own, and the consequences of our sins, the free-will actions of others that damage us, and heredity all could affect us in ways far greater than if we had hidden ourselves under the protection of Almighty God.

While God might not punish us for our actions, He also does not intercede on our behalf when we have put up blocks between us and Him through our willful rebellion and chosen separation. So relational, emotional, and physical problems can be caused by our own choices, or the choices (free will) of others who have done things that affect us.

Other times, we may be negatively affected because of our ignorance. Perhaps we are new in our faith and haven't yet learned of God's covenant blessings for us. A growing Christian will overcome this sort of ignorance with the experience of walking with God, learning about His nature and character, and seeing His will and the truth in His Word as it is confirmed by God's Holy Spirit in us. Scripture tells us that "we have not because we ask not, and when we ask, we ask amiss" or "my people perish because of a lack of knowledge." Thankfully, Jesus promises us that if we continue in His word, we shall "know the truth and the truth will make us free." Only willful ignorance about the things of God is sinful and will hold us back.

Medical science reports that stress lowers our immune system and possibly will allow diseases to fester within us. We usually think stress is caused by external factors such as job, family, finances, disasters, etc. Indeed, these issues do have a cumulative effect on us. But there is also internal stress that is a silent and deadly killer. This internal stress can come from such things in our life as unforgiveness, bitterness, guilt, shame, etc., all caused by our choices that separate us from God's blessings.

If we get closer to God's truth (His will), then the possibilities of receiving His blessings greatly increase. That's the immense benefit of allowing the truth of His word to become your belief. The power lies in closing the gap caused by sin or ignorance.

The information for this Disease Appendix comes from *In His Own Image* by Art Mathias and has been adapted for topics contained in this book.

Praying over Strongholds with This Appendix

1. For each disease listed, prayer topics are specified.

2. Select the emotion or emotions that most readily apply.

3. Go to other topics that you feel are appropriate.

4. You may also need to address deep emotional wounds.

5. When you see the topics "your value" and "forgiveness," quite likely you need to forgive yourself.

6. Observe where anger, bitterness, hatred, rage, and murder are listed. You should also forgive where it is directed. When "self" is prefaced, the emotion is directed at yourself.

7. If specific sins are observed, confessing them and asking for forgiveness of those sins is necessary.

8. Diseases caused by bacteria and viruses will need to be fought off by a strengthened immune system, which is what these scripture verses address.

Remember!
When you go to a topic in this book to pray the scripture, give Jesus permission to search for lies and unbelief and replace them with God's truth.

Acne: anxiety, fear, trust, your value

Acquired Immune Deficiency Syndrome (AIDS): anxiety, fear, forgiveness, rebellion (anger)

Addictions: anxiety, fear, forgiveness, trust, your value

Addison's: guilt, self-hate, your value

Allergies: contentment, fear, feeling forsaken, forgiveness, self-bitterness, your value

Alzheimer's disease: anxiety, forgiveness, guilt, hopelessness, self-hate, your value

Amyloidosis: bitterness, fear, feeling forsaken, forgiveness, your value

Amyotrophic Lateral sclerosis (ALS): anxiety, fear, feeling forsaken, overcoming evil, self-hate, your value

Disease Appendix

Ankylosing Spondylitis: faith, feeling forsaken, forgiveness, guilt, iniquity, self-hate, your value

Aplastic Anemia: feeling forsaken, forgiveness, guilt, your value

Arnold-Chiari Malformation: anger, fear, forgiveness, overcoming evil, rebellion, self-hate, your value

Arthritis: anger, anxiety, fear, forgiveness, self-hate, your value

Asperger's Syndrome: anxiety, forgiveness, guilt, hopelessness, overcoming evil, self-bitterness, your value,

Astrocytoma (brain tumor): iniquity, overcoming evil, self-bitterness, unforgiveness, your value

Attention Deficit Disorder (ADD)/Attention Deficit Hyperactivity Disorder (ADHD): anger, fear, feeling forsaken, forgiveness, overcoming evil, rebellion, your value

Autism: feeling forsaken (self), forgiveness, overcoming evil, rebellion, your value

Bacterial Meningitis: anxiety, fear, feeling forsaken, iniquity

Bechet's Syndrome: fear, forgiveness, guilt, self-hate, your value

Bell's Palsy: anxiety, fear, forgiveness, overcoming evil, self-hate, worry, your value

Benign Prostatic Hyperplasia (enlarged prostate): anger, anxiety, self-bitterness, unforgiveness of sin, worry, your value

Berger's Disease (IgA nephropathy / kidney disorder: guilt, self-hate, unforgiveness, your value,

Bipolar Mood Disorder (Manic-Depression): accepting God's love, anger anxiety, guilt, hopelessness, self-bitterness,

Bursitis: anger, anxiety, fear, forgiveness, injury, self-bitterness, worry, your value

<u>Cancers</u> (bitterness and forgiveness are the central themes)

   Bladder Cancer: anxiety, fear, guilt, trust, unforgiveness, your value

   Bone Cancer: bitterness, faith, fear, feeling forsaken, forgiveness

   Breast Cancer: anxiety, bitterness (bitterness directed toward another woman), faith, fear, forgiveness

   Burkitt's Lymphoma: bitterness, fear, feeling forsaken, forgiveness, iniquity

   Chronic Myeloid Leukemia (CML): anger, anxiety, bitterness, forgiveness, guilt, hopelessness, self-bitterness, your value

   Cervical Cancer: bitterness, overcoming evil, unforgiveness of sin, your value

   Colon Cancer: bitterness, faith, fear, healing

   Hodgkin's Disease: bitterness, faith, feeling forsaken, forgiveness, your value

   Leukemia: bitterness, faith, feeling forsaken, forgiveness, self-bitterness, your value

   Liver Cancer: bitterness, fear, forgiveness, overcoming evil, trust, your value

Lung Cancer: anxiety, bitterness, faith, fear, forgiveness, trust, your value

Multiple Myeloma: anxiety, bitterness, fear, feeling forsaken, forgiveness, trust, self-bitterness, your value

Non-Hodgkin's Lymphoma: anxiety, bitterness, faith, fear, feeling forsaken, forgiveness, guilt, self-bitterness, trust, your value

Ovarian Cancer: bitterness, faith, feeling forsaken, unforgiveness, self-hate, your value

Pancreatic Cancer: anxiety, bitterness, faith, fear, forgiveness, self-bitterness, trust, your value

Prostate Cancer: bitterness, faith, fear, iniquity, unforgiveness

Skin Cancer: bitterness, faith, unforgiveness, your value

Uterine Cancer: bitterness, faith, fear, forgiveness, self-bitterness, your value

Waldenstrom's Macroglobulinemia: bitterness, fear, feeling forsaken, overcoming evil, self-bitterness, unforgiveness

Candidiasis: anxiety, bitterness, faith, feeling forsaken, overcoming evil, unforgiveness, worry

Carpal Tunnel Syndrome: anger, anxiety, faith, fear, self-hate, trust, unforgiveness, your value

Celiac Disease: anxiety, faith, fear, guilt, iniquity, self-hate, your value

Chronic Fatigue: anxiety, fear, guilt, hopelessness, self-hate, your value

Chronic Pain Syndrome: (fear and anxiety increase pain)

Chronic Back Pain: anger, anxiety, faith, fear, strength, worry, your value

Chronic Pelvic Pain: anger, anxiety, guilt/shame, hopelessness, self-bitterness

Pain (psychogenic) without Cause: anxiety, guilt, hate, hopelessness, strength, unforgiveness, your value

Chronic Obstructive Pulmonary Disease (COPD): anxiety, faith, fear, forgiveness, self-hate, trust, your value

Costochondritis: anxiety, fear, forgiveness, guilt, self-bitterness, your value

Crest Syndrome: faith, fear, feeling forsaken, guilt, love, self-hate

Crohn's Disease: anxiety, bitterness, fear (of man), forgiveness, guilt, hopelessness, self-hate

Cushing's Disease: faith, fear (of man), forgiveness, guilt, self-hate, strength, your value

Cystitis (bladder inflammation): anxiety, faith, fear, overcoming evil, self-hate, unforgiveness of sin, your value

Cysts: anxiety, faith, fear, self-bitterness, unforgiveness, your value

Deep Vein Thrombosis (DVT): anger, faith, unforgiveness

Degenerative Disc Disease: anxiety, fear, forgiveness, guilt, hopelessness, self-bitterness, trust, your value

Dementia: anxiety, faith, fear, forgiveness, self-bitterness, your value

Depression: anxiety, forgiveness, guilt, hopelessness, rage, self-bitterness, your value

Dermatitis: anxiety, faith, fear, strength, your value

Diabetes: anxiety, fear, feeling forsaken, forgiveness, guilt, hopelessness, self-hate, your value

Dissociative Disorder (DID) or Multiple Personality Disorder: bitterness, fear, forgiveness, guilt, your value (need for deep healing)

Diffuse Idiopathic Skeletal Hyperostosis: faith, fear, forgiveness, guilt, self-bitterness, your value

Diverticulitis: anger, anxiety, faith, fear, forgiveness

Dyslexia: fear, feeling forsaken, forgiveness, iniquity, rebellion, your value

Dysmenorrhea (menstrual cramps): anxiety, faith, fear, self-hate, unforgiveness, your value

Ear Infections (chronic): faith, fear, feeling forsaken, forgiveness, iniquity, overcoming evil

<u>Eating Disorders</u> (your value)

    Anorexia Nervosa and Bulimia Nervosa: anxiety, fear, forgiveness, hopelessness, self-hate, trust, your value

    Obesity: anxiety, fear, feeling forsaken, forgiveness, guilt, hopelessness, self-bitterness, your value

Eclampsia: anger, faith, fear, feeling forsaken, forgiveness, trust, your value

Endocarditis (nonbacterial): forgiveness, guilt, self-hate, your value

Endometriosis: fear, guilt, self-hate, strength, trust, your value

Environmental Illness (EI): anxiety, faith, fear, feeling forsaken, self-hate, your value

Epilepsy: faith, guilt, overcoming evil

Erectile Dysfunction: anxiety, faith, fear, guilt, hopelessness, self-hate, your value

Essential Tremor: anxiety, fear, hate, overcoming evil, unforgiveness, your value

Fibrocystic Breast Syndrome: forgiveness, iniquity, self-bitterness, your value

Fibromyalgia Syndrome: anxiety, fear, feeling forsaken, forgiveness, hopelessness, self-hate, trust, your value

Flesh Eating Bacteria (Necrotizing Fasciitis): anxiety, faith, fear, overcoming evil, your value

Frigidity (female loss of sexual desire): anger, anxiety, fear, guilt, hopelessness, self-bitterness, your value

Fungal Infections: anxiety, bitterness, fear, forgiveness, overcoming evil

Gallbladder Disease: bitterness, fear, forgiveness, self-bitterness, your value

Gastritis: anxiety, fear, forgiveness, hate, trust, your value

Gingivitis: anxiety, fear, forgiveness, self-hate, your value

Glomerulonephritis: anger, anxiety, fear, trust, unforgiveness, your value

Gout: forgiveness, guilt, self-bitterness, trust, your value

Graves Disease (hyperthyroid): anxiety, faith, fear, forgiveness, guilt, self-hate, your value

Guillain-Barré Syndrome: anxiety, faith, fear, forgiveness, overcoming evil, self-hate, trust, your value

Hair Loss: anxiety, fear, self-hate, unforgiveness, your value

Hashimoto's Disease (hypothyroidism): anxiety, faith, fear, forgiveness, guilt, self-hate, your value

Headache Disorders

Tension Headache: anger, anxiety, bitterness, fear, forgiveness, worry, your value

Migraine Headache: anger, anxiety, fear, forgiveness, guilt, hopelessness, your value

Rebound Headache: anxiety, fear, forgiveness, hopelessness, self-bitterness, trust, your value

Hearing Loss: anxiety, faith, fear, overcoming evil

Heart Disease

Atrial Fibrillation: anxiety, bitterness, fear, forgiveness, guilt, hopelessness, self-hate, worry, your value

Angina: anger, anxiety, fear, forgiveness, guilt, hopelessness, your value

Billowing Mitral Valve Prolapse (MVP): anger, anxiety, fear, forgiveness, guilt, hopelessness, your value

Cardiomyopathy: anxiety, fear, forgiveness, hopelessness, self-hate, trust, your value

Congestive Heart Failure: anger, anxiety, fear, forgiveness, guilt, hopelessness, self-bitterness, your value

Coronary Artery Disease: anxiety, fear, forgiveness, guilt, hopelessness, self-anger, your value

Hepatitis: anxiety, fear, guilt, hate, hopelessness, overcoming evil, your value

Hernia: anger, faith, forgiveness

Herpes Simplex Virus (weak immune system)

Cold Sores and Blisters (Type 1): anxiety, bitterness, fear, forgiveness, stress, your value

Genital Herpes (Type 2): anxiety, bitterness, fear, forgiveness of sin, self-hate, your value

Cytomegalovirus (CMV): anxiety, bitterness, fear, forgiveness of sin, self-hate, your value

Shingles: anxiety, faith, fear

Epstein-Barr Virus (Mononucleosis): anxiety, bitterness, fear, forgiveness, self-hate, your value

High Blood Pressure: anger, anxiety, fear, forgiveness

High Cholesterol: anxiety, faith, fear, guilt, self-anger, unforgiveness, your value

Hives: anxiety, fear

Hyperparathyroidism: anxiety, fear, forgiveness, guilt, hopelessness, self-bitterness, your value

Hypoglycemia: anxiety, fear, feeling forsaken, forgiveness, self-bitterness, trust, your value

Idiopathic Immunologic Thrombocytopenia Purpura (auto-immune blood disorder): fear, feeling forsaken, guilt, hate, love, your value

Infertility: anxiety, fear, forgiveness of sin, guilt, hopelessness, self-hate, trust, your value

Insomnia: anxiety, fear, guilt, hopelessness, overcoming evil, trust, unforgiveness

Insulin Resistance Syndrome: fear, feeling forsaken, forgiveness, hopelessness, self-anger, your value

Interstitial Cystitis (IC): faith, fear, forgiveness, guilt, self-bitterness, trust, your value

Intracranial Hemorrhage (cranial aneurysm): anger, anxiety, fear, forgiveness

Iritis: anxiety, faith, fear, forgiveness, guilt, self-hate, pride, your value

Irritable Bowel Syndrome: anxiety, bitterness, fear, guilt, hopelessness, unforgiveness

Recurrent Abdominal Pain in Children: anxiety, fear, feeling forsaken, trust your value

Kidney Stone: anxiety, faith, fear, feeling forsaken, self-bitterness, your value

Lactose Intolerance: bitterness, fear, feeling forsaken, forgiveness, iniquity, your value

Leaky Gut Syndrome: anxiety, faith, fear, forgiveness, self-hate, your value

Lewy Body Disease: faith, fear, guilt, overcoming evil, self-hate, your value

Lichen Planus: bitterness, faith, guilt, self-hate, your value

Lupus: faith, forgiveness, guilt, self-hate, your value

Lyme Disease: anxiety, faith, fear, forgiveness, guilt, self-hate, your value

Malabsorption: anxiety, fear, forgiveness, your value

Memory Loss: anxiety, fear, worry

Meniere's Disease: anxiety, fear, forgiveness, overcoming evil, self-hate, your value

Menopause: anxiety, fear, feeling forsaken, forgiveness, guilt, resentment, self-hate, worry, your value

Menorrhagia (heavy uterine bleeding): anxiety, fear, forgiveness, guilt, trust, your value

Miscarriage: forgiveness, guilt, self-hate, your value

Mixed Connective Tissue Disease: forgiveness, guilt, self-hate, your value

Multiple Sclerosis: feeling forsaken, forgiveness, guilt, hopelessness, self-hate, trust, your value

Myasthenia Gravis: anxiety, faith, fear, feeling forsaken, forgiveness, self-bitterness, your value

Narcolepsy: anxiety, fear, forgiveness, overcoming evil, self-bitterness, your value

Osteoporosis: anxiety, comfort, fear, forgiveness, guilt, hopelessness, self-bitterness, trust, your value

Pancreatitis: faith, fear, forgiveness, self-bitterness, trust, your value

Parasites: anxiety, fear, taking all thoughts captive

Parkinson's Syndrome: faith, fear, feeling forsaken, hopelessness, iniquity, overcoming evil

Pericarditis (idiopathic): anxiety, faith, fear, forgiveness, guilt, self-hate, your value

Phobic Disorders (fears)

Obsessive Compulsive Disorder: fear, forgiveness, your value

Obsessive Compulsive Personality: fear, forgiveness, your value

Body Dysmorphic Disorder: fear, feeling forsaken, forgiveness, guilt, self-hate, your value

Tourette's Syndrome: anger, fear, forgiveness, your value

Post-Traumatic Stress Disorder (requires deep healing): anxiety, fear, forgiveness, guilt, hopelessness, your value

Acute Stress Disorder: anxiety, fear, forgiveness, guilt, hopelessness, your value

Polycystic Ovarian Syndrome: anger, faith, fear, forgiveness, guilt, strength, your value

Post-Lyme Disease: faith, fear, forgiveness, self-hate, your value

Postpartum Depression: anxiety, fear, guilt, hopelessness, self-hate, unforgiveness, your value (pray these same scripture verses over your child)

Preeclampisa (pregnant women): anger, faith, fear, feeling forsaken, forgiveness, guilt, hopelessness, your value (pray these same scripture verses over your child after birth)

Premenstrual Syndrome: accepting God, anger, anxiety, fear, feeling forsaken, forgiveness, guilt, hopelessness, trust, your value

Psoriasis: faith, fear, feeling forsaken, forgiveness, guilt, self-hate, your value

Pulmonary Fibrosis (idiopathic): faith, feeling forsaken, forgiveness, self-hate, your value

Reflux: anxiety, fear

Reiter's Syndrome: anger, guilt, iniquity, trust, your value

Resting Tremor: anxiety, fear

Restless Leg Syndrome: anxiety, fear, forgiveness, guilt, self-bitterness, strength, your value

Rosacea: anger, anxiety, faith, fear, forgiveness, your value

Reflex Sympathetic Dystrophy (RSD): fear, forgiveness, self-bitterness, your value

Sarcoidosis: feeling forsaken, forgiveness, hate, love, your value

Schizophrenia: discernment, faith, fear, feeling forsaken, forgiveness, overcoming evil, rebellion, self-hate, your value

Scleroderma: faith, forgiveness, guilt, self-hate, your value

Scoliosis: anger, fear, forgiveness, iniquity, rebellion, your value

Sinusitis (chronic): anxiety, fear, feeling forsaken, forgiveness, self-hate, trust, your value

Sjogren's Syndrome: forgiveness, grief, guilt, self-hate, your value

Sleep Apnea: faith, fear, overcoming evil, self-hate, unforgiveness, your value

Stevens Johnson Syndrome: faith, forgiveness, guilt, self-hate, strength, your value

Strabismus: forgiveness, iniquity, overcoming evil, self-hate, your value

Stroke: anger, forgiveness, self-bitterness, your value

Stuttering: fear, forgiveness, self-hate, your value

Suicide: anxiety, fear, forgiveness, guilt, hopelessness, self-hate, your value

Synovitis: faith, fear, forgiveness, guilt, self-hate, your value

Tinnitus: anxiety, faith, fear, overcoming evil

Transient Ischemic Attacks (TIAs): anxiety, faith, fear, forgiveness, self-bitterness, your value

Trigeminal Neuralgia: anxiety, fear, forgiveness, overcoming evil, self-hate, your value

Upper Respiratory Illness: anger, anxiety, fear, feeling forsaken, forgiveness, self-bitterness, your value

Ulcers: anxiety, fear, feeling forsaken, forgiveness, self-bitterness, your value

Ulcerative Colitis: anxiety, feeling forsaken, forgiveness, self-bitterness, your value

Varicose Veins: forgiveness, self-anger, your value

Vitiligo: anxiety, fear, forgiveness, guilt, self-hate, your value

Vulvodynia: faith, fear, unforgiveness of sin

Wegener's Granulomatosis: faith, feeling forsaken, forgiveness, self-anger, trust, your value

Wilson's Syndrome: anxiety, fear, forgiveness, guilt, hopelessness, self-bitterness, your value

About the Author

Neil Elmer has a heart for God and helping others. At a time when Neil needed God the most, he found the Lord's promises through scripture—His Word—the Bible. And he found the Lord's faithfulness through prayer. When Neil began praying scripture, he realized one amazing thing … that it works!

It was only natural that he began sharing scripture with others and encouraged friends and relatives to adopt the idea of praying scripture. Soon, people from across the country were requesting more scripture verses and what began as an idea on a scribble pad became enough material for a book.

It is with a deep sense of humbleness and humilty that the author shares with you "what the Good Doctor ordered" — PreScriptures for Life!

You Can Help Others Find Peace and Comfort!

Share your testimony!

We would like you to email us your testimony on how this book has helped you, a friend, or a relative. Your testimony could be published on www.PreScriptures.com for others to view. So often, testimonies provide motivation and inspiration to help others draw closer to God. Share your testimony today!

We invite you to visit our Web site and participate in our Web-based community!

www.PreScriptures.com

Email us at:

info@PreScriptures.com

Available from
Harvest Day Books

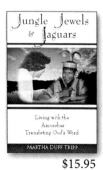

$15.95

Jungle Jewels & Jaguars
Living with the Amueshas Translating God's Word
By Martha Tripp

The true story of a young woman's journey deep into the jungles of Peru to live with the native Amuesha tribe, learn their language, and bring to them the Word of God in their native tongue. This amazing memoir brings us the trials and triumphs of this 23-year Bible translation mission.

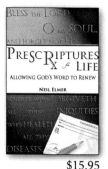

$15.95

PreScriptures for Life
Praying Scriptures: Allowing God's Word to Renew
By Neil Elmer

Prescriptures for Life is about tapping into God's power to overcome obstacles that get in the way of moving forward in life. This user-friendly book provides pertinent Scripture in a topical format—easy to use and share with a friend. Take your prayer life to a deeper level. This handy reference is great for one-on-one personal ministry.

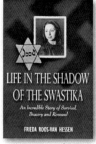

$15.95

Life in the Shadow of the Swastika
An Incredible Story of Survival, Bravery, and Renewal
By Frieda Roos-van Hessen

This powerful, true story recounts the spectacular journey of Frieda as she struggled to survive the Nazi occupation of Holland. As friends and family fell victim to Nazi annihilation, Frieda, along with her friend, Meika, made one death defying escape after another. Experience the emotional rollercoaster as courage, hope, and strength are put to the ultimate test—and salvation of Christ triumphs!

Available from
Harvest Day Books

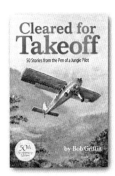

Cleared for Takeoff
50 Stories from the Pen of a Jungle Pilot
50th Anniversary Edition
By Bob Griffin

Veteran missionary aviator, Bob Griffin, shares from his many experiences, beginning with his flight to Ecuador in 1956, where he initiated the aviation program supporting Bible translators. The collection of short stories in this 50th Anniversary Edition are sure to hug your heart and encourage your soul.

$12.95

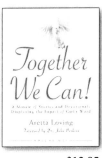

Together We Can!
A Mosaic of Stories and Devotions Displaying the Impact of God's Word
By Aretta Loving

"*Together We Can!* brings us stories about the truth of God's Word, changed lives, miracles, and increased faith. The one thing they all have in common is the power of the Word of God..."
—Dr. John R. Watters
Executive Director Wycliffe International

$12.95

To Place an Order

For additional copies of *PreScriptures for Life*, or for any title by Harvest Day Books, please visit www.ReadingUp.com. Discounts are available for bulk orders to churches, bookstores, and libraries.

Fax orders:	(231)929-1993
Telephone orders:	(231)929-1999
E-mail orders:	orders@bookmarketingsolutions.com
Internet orders:	www.ReadingUp.com

ReadingUp.com

Contact Us

We invite you to visit our Web site!

www.PreScriptures.com

You will find helpful materials for prayer groups, words of encouragement from the author, and testimonies of how God has helped people when they have prayed the scriptures. You may even contribute your own testimony of how praying scripture has helped you in your Christian walk or see how others are providing a prayer ministry to those in need. And much more!

Praying scripture is a grassroots movement, spread mostly by word-of-mouth and one-on-one ministry. Be sure to share it with a friend! Books are available in bulk at discount prices.

Email:	info@PreScriptures.com
Write:	PreScriptures c/o Harvest Day Books 10300 E. Leelanau Ct. Traverse City MI 49684
Web:	www.PreScriptures.com